SECRETS OF
GREAT SKIN

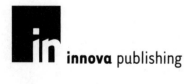
innova publishing

SECRETS OF
GREAT SKIN

THE DEFINITIVE GUIDE TO ANTI-AGING SKIN CARE

DAVID J. GOLDBERG, M.D.
AND EVA M. HERRIOTT, PH.D.

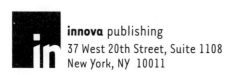

innova publishing
37 West 20th Street, Suite 1108
New York, NY 10011

Secrets of Great Skin

LCCN: 2004107850
ISBN: 0974937320

This book has also been published under the title, *Light Years Younger.*

Published by arrangement with Capital Books, Inc.

Manufactured in the United States of America on acid-free paper.

10   9   8   7   6   5   4   3   2   1

To my patients, whose ever-youthful
spirits continue to inspire me

Contents

Foreword

*T*he blessing (and sometimes the curse) of the high-tech electronic age is that an unlimited amount of information is available, including the latest on health and cosmetic topics. Unfortunately, the amount of information can be overwhelming, confusing, biased, misleading, and even incorrect. The many recent advances that have occurred in understanding the processes involved with aging skin, how to better care for and protect our skin, and how to provide more effective treatment for the effects of aged or sun-damaged skin have served to further confuse everyone. So, how can we accurately evaluate the quality of the information being provided on television talk shows, in newspapers and magazines, and on the Internet?

To the rescue comes Dr. David J. Goldberg and his book, *Secrets of Great Skin: The Definitive Guide to Anti-Aging Skin Care*. It is truly an honor for me to be asked to provide the foreword for this book, written by one of the brightest, most ethical, and most uniquely qualified dermatologists and dermatologic surgeons in our specialty today. It represents an informative approach to skin issues that are of greatest concern to the aging baby boomer population. While this information is based on important scientific concepts, many of which are new, it is written in an enjoyable, easy-to-ready style that makes it understandable and fun.

The book is organized into four parts: Slowing Down the Clock: Beauty Care for the Twenty-first Century; Prevention:

How to Keep Aging in Check; Caring for Your Skin: Break-through Skin Care Techniques for Turning Back the Clock; and Erasing Aging: Advanced Treatments for a More Youthful You.

In part one, Dr. Goldberg explains how and why our skin ages, the differences in aging between men and women, and the effects of smoking on our skin. He also introduces the new concept of "cosmeceuticals," those myriad agents available without a pre-scription that are not only just cosmetics, but that also contain active ingredients that can protect the skin or improve its appear-ance. In part two, Dr. Goldberg explains the effects of sunlight protection, diet, exercise, hormones, and stress on the aging process. Part three provides many useful suggestions on how to maintain healthy-looking skin at any age, and how to stay look-ing young using topical home products. Part four provides a use-ful guide on new methods and treatments to preserve youthful-looking skin and on what you should do if your skin already suf-fers from the effects of aging. The short "sidebar" discussions and "Ask the Doctor" sections serve to clarify key points for the reader. This innovative style, coupled with the inclusion of refer-ences, distinguish this book from any others on the topic. It is a pleasure for me to recommend this book as the definitive guide. It is presented in an unbiased, scientific, yet readable format for all who are interested in learning about the latest information on the causes, prevention, and improvement of aging skin.

—Ronald G. Wheeland, M.D.

Past President
American Academy of Dermatology

Past President
American Society for Lasers in Medicine and Surgery

Acknowledgments

A very special thanks goes to our agent, Joelle Delbourgo, for contributing her considerable insight and savvy to the conception of this book. Also a deeply felt thank you to media consultant Dean Draznin, without whose vision and creativity this book would not have seen the light of day.

Dr. Goldberg: I would like to extend my appreciation to my scientific colleagues, who continue to inspire me to delve more deeply into the exciting field of anti-aging skin care, especially to Perry Robins, M.D. and Ronald Wheeland, M.D., whose guidance has played a pivotal role in my career.

In addition, a special thanks goes to all my patients and staff at both Skin Laser & Surgery Specialists of New York and New Jersey and New York's Mount Sinai School of Medicine.

Eva M. Herriott: Thank you to my husband, Scott, for his constant support and great companionship, and to my enlightened community of friends who continue to enrich my life in more ways than they will ever know. Also special thanks to Jim Karpen and Bryan Aubrey.

Last but not least, we would like to thank our editors, Judy Karpinski and Judy Coughlin, for their sure hand in orchestrating the final stages of the book and masterfully keeping track of all the little details.

Introduction

When you think of the face of aging, two images might come to mind. You may picture the furrowed, pasty, grandmother-like face most of us associate with old age. You may also think of the stretched, artificial facial features of women who have undergone extensive cosmetic surgery in their struggle to slow the onslaught of aging.

Well, here's good news. Thanks to recent breakthroughs in our knowledge of the skin and how it ages, you no longer have to choose between resigning yourself to the ravages of aging or enduring great physical and financial expense to repair its damages. Women today have access to many more choices than ever before for taking years off their appearance—without cosmetic surgery. Aging need no longer be a slow, inevitable decline of appearance and bodily functions. Instead, it can be a time of gratification and enjoyment, a time to reap and express the wisdom and maturity you have accumulated.

Whether you are reluctantly inching toward the age when those first fine lines morph into deep crow's-feet or are already well into it, you have lots of company. The demographics of this country are changing rapidly, to the tune of more than 75 million baby boomers entering middle age over the next decade. Sandwiched between Generation X and the ailing Generation R_X, this boisterous cohort has never been one to accept the status quo of any phase of life. Middle age is proving to be no exception. As more and more boomers slide into and through middle age, they are transforming our notions of aging and shaping numerous trends in their refusal to accept the declines of aging. Active retirement, age management, anti-aging medicine, and an increased focus on healthy lifestyle habits are just a few of the cultural phenomena forged by boomers in their rejection of the conventional trappings of aging. Personal appearance is no exception—boomers are determined to slow the clock of aging, preferably taking it back a ticktock or two.

So if you are one of the numerous middle-aged boomers who are increasingly unhappy with the face staring back at you in your mirror—or one of the many over-thirty women or men who realize that one can never start too early to counteract age-related physical decline—time is on your side. We live in an exciting age. The last ten years have brought an explosion of new skin care treatments that curb the progression of aging, many of which have appeared within just the past couple of years. Our knowledge of the body and how to enhance our health, well-being, and appearance has never been greater. There are more opportunities than ever before for remaining radiant and good-looking to a ripe old age, while avoiding the pitfalls and pain of the one-size-fits-all approach of cosmetic surgery techniques.

As people live longer, the need to adopt techniques for making the most of one's appearance at all stages of life is increasing. Life expectancy has gone up dramatically over the past century, and both women and men live longer, healthier lives than ever before. A woman born in the nineteenth century could expect to live until she was forty-eight; today her life expectancy is seventy-nine. The average nineteenth-century man lived until the age of forty-six; today men, on average, live until age seventy-two.

As the proportion of the population attaining old age increases, there is a growing disparity between the values of society, which equate youthfulness with beauty, success, and desirability, and the marks left by the advance of time. Fortunately, the many exciting new anti-aging beauty treatments that have appeared within the last decade hold great promise to enable us to enjoy all facets of life to the fullest and stay socially and sexually active to a ripe old age.

The biggest barrier most people face in taking full advantage of the many new age-erasing skin care products and treatments is lack of information. Many people are simply not aware of all the new skin care solutions now available; others have heard of them but don't know how to choose or combine treatments to create the most complete and powerful anti-aging regimen. Still others are wary, because they have heard stories of botched treatments that create beauty problems instead of solving them.

In this book we show you how to take advantage of recent breakthroughs in our knowledge of the skin and its care to slow the advance of aging and look younger than your age—at any age. You will learn:

- How to harness the skin's own powerful regenerating abilities to maintain a youthful appearance well into middle age.
- How to protect yourself against the one single factor that more than anything else causes aging of the skin.
- How to take advantage of the many exciting breakthroughs in skin care products to restore the fresh glow of your skin and reduce fine lines and wrinkles.
- How to separate products that really work from those that do not and how to choose the products that fit your particular needs.

- How to address aging at the deepest layers of the skin, where the changes that precede the visible signs of aging take place.
- How to take full advantage of the numerous, noninvasive breakthrough anti-aging treatments that have emerged within the last few years.

In short, this book lays out all the information you will need to make the transition to maturity without saying good-bye to your good looks. Join us as we explore the exciting new knowledge and techniques now available to help you create a complete and powerful, noninvasive anti-aging program to maximize your appearance and well-being.

PART I

Slowing Down the Clock:
Beauty Care for the Twenty-first Century

CHAPTER 1

Options for Aging

Who is to say that life is fair? The one time in your life when you enjoy smooth, glowing, perfect skin is the time when you appreciate it the least: between the age of birth and adolescence. Then the golden teenage years dawn, and suddenly you care a lot about how you look—just in time for the hormonal roller coaster of puberty to inflict its devastation on your skin. Many people are well into their twenties before their skin recovers from the hormonal challenges of adolescence.

Then, somewhere between thirty and forty-five, the painful realization dawns that by some cruel twist of fate, you are getting older. This sudden insight bursts on our awareness when denial no longer suffices to disregard the dreaded signature signs of aging—the brown spots, droops, drops, crinkles, creases, crow's-feet, folds, and furrows that signal the end of youth.

The groundwork for many of these changes, however, was laid long before they appeared, while your cheeks were still glowing with the freshness of youth and the thought that you would ever get older was the furthest thing from your mind. The majority of the age-related changes we see in the skin over time are the cumulative results of the habits we have entertained every day of our lives. Seemingly innocuous habits, such as how much time you spend outside, how much sleep you get at night, how healthy a diet you eat, and how much exercise you get, have a major influence on the way your skin looks from your mid-thirties and onward.

This is actually good news, because it means that while some components of skin aging are inevitable, others can be avoided entirely or at least postponed. By developing greater awareness of your skin, how to take care of it and protect it, you can slow down the progression of aging and take years off your face. Even if your skin already exhibits advanced signs of aging, you can reverse much of the damage by taking proper care of your skin and using the appropriate age-erasing treatments.

And it's never too late to start.

Not All 35+-Year-Olds Are Created Equal: Factors that Influence the Rate at Which Your Skin Ages

Scientists divide skin aging into two categories—*intrinsic* and *extrinsic* aging. Intrinsic aging includes the age-related changes that you cannot control. These originate predominantly in genetic factors and unfold over time at a predetermined pace. Extrinsic aging, on the other hand, is caused by factors that you can control. As you will learn throughout this book, you can do numerous things to avoid or even reverse the damage wrought by extrinsic aging.

INTRINSIC AGING: THE KEY PLAYERS

Genetic Factors. When you think of intrinsic aging, think hered-ity. The processes of intrinsic aging are the same for each indi-vidual, but your genetic legacy dictates the rate at which they unfold. The way your parents' skin aged will give you good clues to how your own skin will age. If one or both of your parents enjoyed youthful skin to an advanced age, you may well be for-tunate enough to have inherited the same characteristics.

Hormonal Changes. One of the most dramatic changes in a woman's appearance takes place in the years surrounding meno-pause. The drop in estrogen levels associated with menopause is well known to weaken the bones and increase a woman's risk of contracting osteoporosis. However, reduced estrogen affects the health of the skin as well, causing a substantial loss of collagen, an important protein that makes up most of the skin's supportive structure. The result is the proliferation of wrinkles and sagging skin often seen in postmenopausal women.

Cellular Decline. Although the visible signs of aging are appar-ent in the furrows, sags, and wrinkles of an older face, the pro-cesses of aging actually originate at a microscopic level, i.e., on the level of each individual cell. Skin aging is the result of a cumulative loss of numerous functions at the cellular level, which decreases the cells' capacity to perform the metabolic and regenerating activities that uphold the health of the skin.

EXTRINSIC AGING: THE MAIN OFFENDERS

Extrinsic aging is a far more powerful factor in the aging process than the time-related decay in biological functions associated with intrinsic aging. Fortunately, most of the factors that induce extrinsic aging are largely avoidable.

Mostly for Men

 Ever wonder why men seem to have fewer wrinkles than their female counterparts of similar age? Male skin ages differently from female skin, because its structure is different in a number of ways. To begin with, men have—no pun intended—thicker skin. On average, male skin is 25 percent thicker than female skin. The top layer of the skin, where wrinkles are most apparent, is thicker and hence less prone to wrinkles. In addition, male skin has higher collagen content, the protein that forms part of the skin's supportive structure. Last, the oil glands in male skin excrete greater quantities of oil, which create a thicker, protective film on the surface of the skin and guard against moisture loss and excessive dryness.

The collagen content of male skin declines much more gradually than that of women. Whereas women experience a dramatic decline in collagen content and consequent thinning of the skin at the onset of menopause, the collagen in male skin breaks down gradually, at a rate of about 1 percent per year. And since men have much more collagen to begin with, they typically do not develop the mesh of fine lines and wrinkles that often emerge as a woman's skin loses its collagen support.

Excessive Sun Exposure. Of all the influences that cause premature aging, no single one is as important as sunlight. In our time and age, damage caused by excessive exposure to the sun is without a doubt *the* leading cause of skin aging. In fact, researchers estimate that skin damage induced by the ultraviolet rays of the sun is responsible for up to 80 percent of the skin's aging.

One of the main reasons that sunlight is so harmful to the skin is that ultraviolet (UV) radiation triggers free radicals production in the skin. Free radicals are molecules that are missing an electron and hence are in a state of chemical disequilibrium. To restore their balance, they turn into little molecular-sized "Pacmans," gobbling up electrons from surrounding molecules and, in the process, wreaking havoc at the cellular level of the body.

Free radical damage is serious business. Excess free radical production is thought to increase the risk of numerous chronic diseases, including such leading killers as heart disease, stroke, and cancer. When free radicals are produced in excess in the skin, they attack the collagen in the skin, causing it to lose its resilience and strength and accelerating the appearance of wrinkles.

Most of the sun damage that induces premature aging typically happens in the early part of our lives, but the results don't show up until years later. For many people, early-life sun damage is a ticking time bomb that is set off once they enter their late thirties or forties. Fortunately, as we see in later chapters, there are many ways not only to protect yourself against further sun damage, but to actually reverse the damage the sun might already have wrought on your skin.

Smoking. The term "smoker's face" was coined to characterize the maze of creases, crinkles, and deep grooves, and the dull, lifeless complexion one often sees on the faces of longtime smokers. If you don't care that much about how you age, go ahead—smoke to your heart's content! Apart from spending long hours in the sun, there is no better way to make sure your skin ages prematurely.

The list of the ways in which smoking affects the skin is long, but it can be summed up in one word: *choking.* Smoking decreases the flow of oxygen to the skin by as much as 30 percent. Cigarette smoke causes the fine blood vessels in the dermis to constrict, cutting off the nutrient supply the skin needs for constant self-regeneration and blocking the removal of waste products. As a result, the skin's natural functions are compromised, and the skin begins to look gray and dull.

Spotlight on Research

DOES PASSIVE SMOKING
CAUSE PREMATURE AGING?
Even if you don't smoke, there is evidence that the
health of your skin will be negatively affected if you
spend a lot of time in the company of people who do. In a study of
one hundred people, both active and "passive" smokers—i.e., people
who had never smoked, but had lived or worked with heavy smokers for twenty years—showed similar deterioration of the skin.
Active and "passive" smokers had the same degree of skin dryness
and damage to the protective barrier of the epidermis. The
researchers concluded that exposure to smoke might be as harmful
to the skin as exposure to the sun.

Smoking also triggers free radical production in the body, upset-
ting the delicate balance of bodily tissues and organs and causing
similar damage to the skin as UV radiation. In fact, the combination of excessive sun exposure and smoking is a deadly cocktail
for your skin and a surefire way to induce premature aging.

Air Pollution. Airborne toxic waste products affect the skin in
much the same way as cigarette smoke. Air pollutants restrict the
flow of oxygen and nutrients to the skin and, in addition, trigger
excess free radical production. Free radicals are always present in
the body; they are a byproduct of normal metabolic activity, and
the body has a series of built-in mechanisms for neutralizing
them before they go on a rampage in the cellular environment.
However, external influences, such as sunlight, smoke, and
industrial pollution, can tip the balance of free radicals in the
body and cause them to increase beyond the body's capacity to
inactivate them.

The effect of free radical damage on the skin and how to counteract it is one of the newest and most exciting areas of research in dermatology today. When it comes to managing the aging process, understanding free radicals and how to neutralize them is a key step. In later chapters, we show you how to control or even reverse free radical damage.

Wear and Tear. Wear and tear is another source of extrinsic aging. The expression lines that emerge when you smile, frown, or lift your eyebrows create a constant mechanical challenge to the skin tissue in those areas. Over time, this shows up in your face as smile lines around your mouth and eyes, vertical furrows between your brows, or horizontal lines on your forehead. Similarly, if you sleep on your side with your face against a pillow year after year, the pressure of the skin against the pillow will cause creases that eventually become permanent. Such lines are less likely to emerge if you sleep on your back.

Your skin can also be damaged if you are exposed to excessive heat or cold. If you live in a place where the winters are harsh and cold, your skin will be challenged not only by the cold temperature, but also by the dry air common during the winter. In addition, people who spend a lot of time around the heat emitted from furnaces, stoves, or ovens, such as bakers or cooks, often suffer from premature aging of the skin.

Excessive use of harsh soaps, detergent-based cleansers, or cosmetic products that are too strong for your skin is another source of extrinsic aging. Such products may cause irritation or inflammation of the top layer of the skin, damaging it and accelerating its deterioration.

Lifestyle habits. Numerous elements of your daily routine exert a powerful influence on the appearance of your skin, including your eating habits, how much alcohol you consume, how much sleep you get, the degree of stress to which you are exposed, and the amount and type of exercise you engage in. Poor lifestyle habits affect the whole body and, as a consequence the skin as well, where they typically show up as a dull, sallow, uneven, and prematurely wrinkled complexion. Healthy habits, on the other hand, can increase your well-being, prevent the onset of disease, and slow the progression of aging in your body as well as your skin. In later chapters, you learn how to introduce some simple daily behaviors that have the potential to do more for your skin than almost anything else you can do.

The Many Faces of Beauty

If you are concerned about slowing the advance of time, you are not alone. The desirability of beauty is a universal feature of human life. The standards of beauty may differ from culture to culture, but the search for beauty crosses cultural and historical barriers. Many of today's common beauty care techniques have been with us for thousands of years. Women in ancient cultures performed dermabrasion, or skin resurfacing, using salt, pumice, ground grains, bone, and horn. They also applied numerous exfoliating substances, such as peels made of botanical extracts, animal fats, metals, or food substances containing acids. Queen Cleopatra is said to have used the lactic acid in donkey's milk to retain the flawless complexion that helped woo the mighty Caesar.

From the perspective of modern psychology, our universal quest for beauty is not just an expression of vanity; it makes good sense. Research has shown that individuals who are considered physically attractive enjoy considerable social advantages. In her book, *Survival of the Prettiest,* psychologist Nancy Etcoff of Harvard Medical School notes that beautiful individuals are deemed to have more positive personality characteristics and life experiences. Attractive individuals tend to get preferential treatment in social interactions; people are likely to consider them more confident and more intelligent and act more kindly toward them. In one study, for example, researchers showed photos of women to seventy-five college men and asked them to pick the woman they would be most likely to do an unselfish act for. The acts suggested included donating blood to the woman, moving furniture for her, lending her money, swimming a mile to save her, donating a kidney, and rescuing her from a burning building. Invariably, the men volunteered to do such altruistic acts for one of the more attractive women. The one notable exception to the many charitable deeds they would happily engage in was lending the woman money!

According to Etcoff, beauty confers elite status. Good-looking individuals tend to do better in the job market and earn higher salaries. People are more likely to be persuaded by the opinions of attractive individuals and to yield to them in arguments. We project all sorts of positive qualities on beautiful individuals, expecting them to perform better in their work, enjoy more harmonious and fulfilling marriages, and be more healthy, well-adjusted, and happy.

In turn, beautiful people tend to be more confident and assertive. Research demonstrates that this might be in part because they are affected by the positive feedback they receive from the environment. This was evidenced in a study in which researchers gave a group of men photos of a woman and told them to call her as a potential date. Some men received a photo of a beautiful woman, others received a photo of a plain woman. In reality, however, only the photos differed—the men all called the same woman. The men who thought the woman was beautiful were more cordial, forthcoming, and positive toward her during the phone conversation than the men who thought she was plain. The woman, in turn, responded in a much more animated and confident way when she talked with the men who thought she was pretty than when she talked with the men who thought she was plain. The woman did not know that the men had been shown different pictures of her. She reacted unconsciously to the different attitudes the men projected toward her in the conversation.

While it is useful to be aware of the social advantages and enhanced self-esteem conferred by an attractive appearance, relying on too narrow a definition of beauty can be counterproductive. As the old cliché goes, beauty is more than skin deep. A person's appearance plays a big role in the first impression we have of that person, but obviously numerous additional factors are involved in forming a long-lasting opinion of someone. Many fascinating, competent, and interesting people are not beautiful in the classical sense. Rather, they are attractive because of the charm, confidence, energy, vitality, and charisma they exude. Conversely, the stereotype of the blonde "bimbo," is an expression of society's contempt for beauty that is hollow and does not go beyond surface appearance.

In short, appearance isn't everything. While making the most of your appearance certainly is inherently satisfying, there is no need to let concerns about your appearance dominate your life and cause you to lose touch with the deeper and more important aspects of your personality and identity. Keep in mind that happiness and contentment are the best beauty remedies; getting too hung up on your appearance is counterproductive.

The New Beauty Specialists

At this point, we would like to introduce you to one of your most important resources in curbing the effects of aging: a cosmetic dermatologist. Cosmetic dermatology focuses primarily on nonaggressive, safe approaches to improving the skin and its appearance. Cosmetic dermatology emerged as an active medical

Spotlight on Research

IS THE APPEAL OF BEAUTY AN INBORN TRAIT? A number of researchers argue that beauty has universal appeal because it is hard-wired into our psyche as part of our genetic heritage. According to this theory, a smooth, clear complexion, symmetrical features, and thick, beautiful hair are signs of health and hence of reproductive potential. In short, the appeal of beauty may well be part of a biological adaptation that draws us toward the members of the opposite sex who are most likely to ensure survival of our genetic material.

According to psychologist Judith Langlois, professor of developmental psychology at the University of Texas at Austin, even babies appear to exhibit universal beauty preferences. In one study, Langlois asked adults to rate slides of people's faces by their degree of attractiveness. Next, Langlois showed the faces to three- and six-month-old babies and monitored their responses. The babies looked longer at the faces that the adults had rated as attractive, regardless of whether the faces were male, female, Caucasian, African-American, or Asian-American. In short, recognition of beauty might not just be something we are taught as we grow up, but rather a universal, inborn feature.

specialty only very recently, yet today, it is one of the most prolific areas of medical research. Wedding modern medical knowledge and technologies with esthetic concerns, research in this field has spearheaded development of numerous noninvasive skin care treatments over the past decade. As a result, it is now possible to take years off your appearance without the pain and expense typically associated with plastic surgery.

Although some people use the term *cosmetic dermatology to* include cosmetic surgery, it is preferable to make a distinction between the two, because their methods and techniques are somewhat different. Cosmetic surgery techniques are still in much demand, yet many consumers do not feel entirely comfortable with them, because they are invasive and the results can be artificial-looking. As a result, cosmetic surgery has a mixed reputation in today's society. People who undergo extensive cosmetic surgery to hold on to their youthful looks may become the butt of jokes. As David Letterman once quipped when then-Vice President Al Gore appeared on Letterman's television show: "Whenever you have a big deal like the Vice President on the show, my God, security is tight. Security tonight is tighter than Joan Rivers' face. It's unbelievable!"

Surgical techniques such as facelifts and dermabrasion have numerous other limitations. Dermabrasion can produce unflattering pigmentation in people with dark or brown skin. Facelifts and other plastic surgery procedures are expensive and, as with many other types of surgery, involve a great deal of discomfort.

With the advances in cosmetic dermatology, a happy middle ground has become available. The marriage of medicine, science, and modern technology is producing unprecedented knowledge of the skin and its care. The last ten years in particular have seen an explosion of new skin care treatments that counteract the progression of aging. Many of these advances have been made within just the past couple of years. Women can now benefit from such breakthroughs in anti-aging skin care as:

- Widespread introduction of the so-called *cosmeceuticals*, whose ability to reverse skin aging and reduce wrinkles is backed by solid scientific research
- Proliferation of topical antioxidants and the potential they hold for addressing aging at the deepest layers of the skin, where the changes that precede the visible signs of aging take place

- New and minimally invasive treatments for fine lines and lackluster skin
- Gentle treatments that stimulate new collagen production, avoiding wrinkles before they develop
- Breakthrough therapies for reversing sun damage, including noninvasive treatments such as "lunchtime lasers," microdermabrasion and Intense Pulsed Light™ (IPL) therapy
- New skin-perfecting treatments for wrinkles, age spots, and other age-related complaints that do not involve prolonged healing time and significant risk of complications

Becoming an Informed Consumer

There is a downside to the rapid progress of anti-aging skin care over the past decade. Changes are happening so fast that it can be hard for consumers — and regulators — to keep up. Cosmetic companies are quick to capitalize on new advances in our knowledge of skin and the factors that increase or slow its aging, and it can be hard to ascertain the medical facts behind the enthusiastic marketing claims.

More often than not, skin care products are touted to contain one or several miracle ingredients that magically sweep away wrinkles and restore the skin to its youthful characteristics. Vitamins, minerals, enzymes, antioxidants, hormones, or natural "bioactive" ingredients derived from plants, the sea, the earth, or even oxygen are just a sampling of the many so-called miracle substances that promise to melt away the years. Typically such substances do prove to have important health benefits in one context or other. The problem with crossover claims is that often there is little evidence that such ingredients will have any effect on the skin whatsoever.

Similarly, as more affordable and far less intrusive laser treatments are increasing in popularity, the prospect of easy money has lured a host of poorly trained practitioners to this still relatively unregulated field. In a number of states, even dentists, obstetricians, and family doctors with minimal training and practice now offer laser surgery. The uninformed consumer, in short, faces some very real hazards when contemplating laser surgery. Lasers are potent tools, and, in the hands of the novice user, they can wreak considerable damage on the skin and cause burns and scarring.

In this scenario, it is no wonder that many consumers feel overwhelmed by the conflicting information with which they are constantly bombarded. In this book, we show you how to sort the medical facts from the marketing hype and help you to understand the many important developments taking place in anti-aging skin care. In addition, we give you the tools to determine which skin care products really work and which products are most suitable for your skin type. We also give you a guide to the many breakthrough anti-aging treatments that have emerged on the market within the last few years.

There are more possibilities available than ever before for taking control of your own aging process. The following chapters lay out the knowledge and tools you need to take advantage of the many powerful treatments available to help you extend the number of years during which you enjoy beautiful and glowing skin.

CHAPTER 2

Why Does My Skin Age, and What Can I Do about It?

*T*he drama of aging—at least the visible parts of it—is played out almost entirely on the skin. For better or worse, the surface of the skin forms the center stage of aging, the place where our journey through time is indelibly etched. With advancing age, bodily functions become less efficient—cell turnover slows down, hormone levels decrease, the kidneys filter waste less effectively, the heart grows weaker, and so on. Innocuous at first, these small changes add up and eventually become evident in our appearance—the texture of the skin changes, the complexion becomes more yellow or uneven, wrinkles appear in increasing numbers.

As we saw in the last chapter, however, aging of the skin is not a fixed process, nor is it an inevitable, predetermined decline; it is highly modifiable. Each of us can contribute to our own successful aging, not just in terms of appearance, but in overall energy and zest for life. There is a happy convergence between the health needs dictated by the body and the desire to stay youthful

SECRETS OF GREAT SKIN

and good-looking for as long as possible. The best way to maintain not only your good looks, but your youthfulness, zest for life, and vitality as well is to take full advantage of the many recent advances in our knowledge about the body and the factors that enhance its health. True anti-aging beauty care is not about buying potions and lotions that will magically restore your complexion to its youthful best, although these certainly have their value. It is about working with your body to stay in optimum health while making prudent use of noninvasive anti-aging treatments to enhance your appearance.

To get a complete understanding of the many ways in which you can counteract the pervasive deterioration of the skin triggered by the advance of aging, it is important to first gain insight into the structure and functions of the skin and how these are affected by the aging process. This chapter discusses how aging unfolds in the skin and what you can do to slow its progression.

The Skin—A Primer

The skin is not just a surface mantle that protects your body from the harsh influences of the environment; it is a vital part of the body and a large, highly versatile organ that performs a number of life-sustaining tasks. In fact, the skin is so important that if it is damaged over a large area and loses its ability to function—as sometimes happens in burn victims—a person is not likely to survive.

Your skin works hard every minute of the day to maintain the body's equilibrium. It protects the body from environmental influences and supports its performance in numerous ways. Taking good care of your skin and shielding it from influences that might impair its functions is not just a matter of retaining your good looks; it makes good sense for your long-term health and well-being as well.

Did You Know That . . . ?

- The skin is the largest organ of the body. In an average woman, the skin weighs close to six pounds, in men, an average of nine pounds.
- The thickness of the skin is 0.1 mm in most places, but it is highly variable. The skin is thinnest around the eyes and thickest on the soles of the feet, where it is 0.8 to 1.4 mm thick.
- The skin renews itself constantly: new skin cells are formed at the deeper levels of the skin and travel up to the surface of the skin in a twenty-eight-day cycle.
- The skin's appearance depends on the health of the top layer, the epidermis, and the state of tissues in the deeper layers of the skin.
- Through its sweat glands, the skin plays a key role in regulating the body's temperature. The average person has 2.5 million sweat ducts distributed throughout the body, with the highest concentration under the arms, on the forehead, and on the palms and soles.
- We constantly lose moisture through the sweat ducts, even when we're not obviously perspiring. The minimum amount of perspiration per day is about half a quart, but with excessive perspiration, a person can lose up to ten quarts of moisture in a day.

Whereas the skin may look like a simple, thin layer of tissue, it is, in fact, a complex, multilayered organ (see figure 2.1). The skin consists of three main layers, the *epidermis*, the *dermis*, and the *subcutaneous* fat layer. The epidermis is the outermost layer of the skin, which forms the primary protective coating of the body. Its topmost layer is known as the *stratum corneum*, the "horny layer." This is a thin, tough layer of dead skin cells that acts as our outer "hide." The second layer of skin, the dermis, is the skin's control center. It contains all the vital components that keep the skin nourished, strong, and healthy. It also houses the

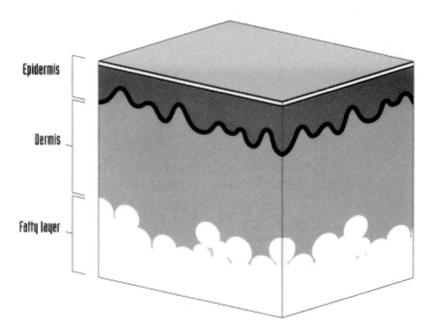

Figure 2.1 The layers of skin.

supportive structures that keep the skin resilient and plump. The third layer, the subcutaneous tissue, is a layer of fat beneath the dermis. It acts as a protective, insulating layer between the surface of the skin and the inner organs and helps the body conserve heat energy.

THE SKIN'S PROTECTIVE MANTLE: THE EPIDERMIS

The primary function of the epidermis is to protect the body from the impact of the environment. The epidermis shields the tender tissues of the body from the harmful rays of the sun, the trauma of extreme cold and heat, and the drying influence of the wind. The body consists of more than 90 percent water, and the epidermis forms a vital waterproof barrier that protects the body against excessive moisture loss and dehydration.

The epidermis also constitutes an important component of the body's immune defense, providing a multilayered shield against environmental pathogens. The deeper levels of the skin discharge a natural oil that is secreted as a thin film on top of the epidermis, creating a slightly acidic environment that inhibits microbe growth. The uppermost layer of the epidermis — the dense, impenetrable band known as the stratum corneum — forms a mechanical barrier against infective microorganisms. If foreign agents such as bacteria, fungi, or yeasts do succeed in getting past these first two levels of defense, the deeper layers of the epidermis contain different types of immune system cells that will attack and immobilize the intruders.

THE SKIN'S SUPPORT CENTER: THE DERMIS

Located just beneath the epidermis, the dermis constitutes about 90 percent of the skin's mass and is the seat of most of the skin's vital functions. The dermis provides the infrastructure and support system of the skin, and its resilient structures protect the body from knocks and bumps. In addition, components of the dermis play an important role in regulating body temperature and transmitting sensory sensations such as touch, heat, cold, and pain.

Of particular relevance for our discussion are the supportive and strength-giving fibers in the dermis, which give the skin its plumpness, resilience, and bounce. In the same way that our skeletal frame creates the supportive structure that upholds the body, the dermis contains fibrous structures that prop up and reinforce the skin. This "skeletal structure" of the skin is made up of two proteins — *collagen* and *elastin* (see figure 2.2).

The collagen and elastin fibers are not rigid like the bony structure of the skeleton. Rather, they are like springs in a mattress — they give the skin bounce and provide a strong, spongy padding that acts as a shock absorber against injury from falls, bumps, and

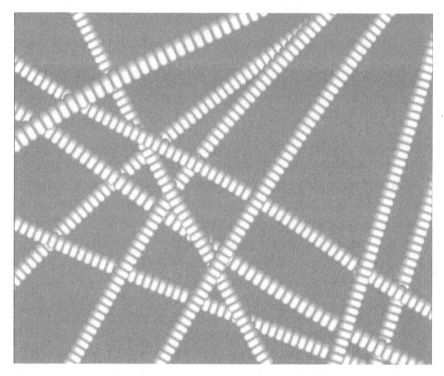

Figure 2.2 Collagen Bundles. *Collagen proteins linked together in bundles constitute the supportive structure of not only the skin, but of most types of soft tissue, including muscles, tendons, and cartilage.*

knocks. The collagen and elastin fibers also hold the structures of the body together and contribute to the shape and form of the body.

Collagen bundles are surrounded by a jellylike material, typically referred to as the *ground substance*. The ground substance acts like a sponge; it absorbs and retains a thick cushion of water, which helps to moisturize the skin and create a protective cushion that insulates the collagen bundles and preserves their resilience. The ground substance is composed primarily of proteins, called *glycosaminogylcans* (GAGs), or *glyoproteins* for short. Glycoproteins can retain up to a thousand times their weight in water and function as a natural hydrator in the skin. One of the main GAGs is *hyaluronic acid,* which can attract and bind consid-

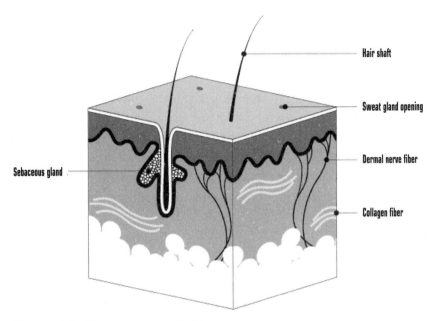

Hair shaft

Sweat gland opening

Dermal nerve fiber

Sebaceous gland

Collagen fiber

Figure 2.3 Components of skin.

erable amounts of water. It acts as a natural moisturizing agent, giving the skin its smooth, supple, and reflective quality.

Apart from its supportive structure, the dermis also contains a number of infrastructure components that provide nourishment to the epidermis. The dermis is packed with lymph channels and with tiny blood vessels that transport oxygen, vitamins, chemicals, and other nutrients needed to regenerate the epidermis. The metabolism of the epidermis in turn produces waste products, which are picked up and carried away by the mesh of blood vessels and lymph channels that pervade the dermis.

The oil glands, or *sebaceous glands,* are another key component of the dermis. They secrete a thin, oily film, referred to as *sebum,* that lies like a protective mantle on the epidermis. As you can see in figure 2.3, the sebaceous glands are located next to the hair follicles at the base of the skin's hair shafts. The hair shaft provides a natural passageway through which the sebum can travel to the surface of the skin.

Finally, the dermis contains a number of independent organs, which are responsible for separate physiological functions. The *sweat glands* play a key role in controlling body temperature. When we perspire, the moisture released by the sweat glands evaporates from the surface of the body, causing heat loss and cooling the body down. Sweating also provides a means of removing waste products and acids from the body. In addition, the dermis is packed with numerous, tiny *nerve endings.* Some of these are responsible for our sense of touch, while others detect pressure or inform the brain about sensations of pain, heat, or cold.

THE SKIN'S CUSHION: THE SUBCUTANEOUS FAT LAYER

The subcutaneous layer of the skin is one area where fat is good. Located beneath the dermis, this deepest part of the skin consists primarily of fat cells, which are organized together into *fat lobules.* When healthy, this layer helps give the skin the plumped-out, smooth, and wrinkle-free complexion of youth.

Like the dermis, the subcutaneous layer contains collagen and elastin fibers and houses blood vessels, nerves, and lymph channels, which are generally larger than those in the dermis. This component of the skin forms a layer of insulation, which helps the body conserve heat. It also acts as a protective cushion for the dermis and for the muscle, bone, and cartilage tissues below the skin.

How the Skin Ages

Aging of the skin consists of a gradual breakdown of numerous different structures and functions. In fact, more than fifty factors are at work in the age-related deterioration of the skin. The good news is that, as a consequence, there is not just one way to counteract skin aging; there are many ways you can enhance the health and youthful appearance of your body's external covering.

Over the past few decades, our knowledge of the factors that accelerate or slow skin's aging has increased vastly. Transformation of the skin over time is a fascinating process that is played out in all three layers of the skin. Wrinkles, age spots, thinning skin, a yellowish or dull complexion, loss of elasticity, droops, sags, grooves, furrows — you name it — they are all the end result of a long series of tiny changes, most of which start as early as your twenties.

Although the signs of aging are apparent at the epidermal level, the health of the dermis and the subcutaneous tissue has an equal, if not greater, impact on the smoothness and radiance of your complexion and the rate at which the signs of aging emerge. So let's journey through the layers of the skin as they are altered with the advance of time. As you gain insight into the age-related changes that emerge in each of the three main layers of skin, you will develop a deeper understanding of how and why different anti-aging treatments work and which ones might be most suitable for your particular needs.

AGE-RELATED CHANGES IN THE EPIDERMIS

Slower Cell Reneal. The epidermis constantly replaces itself. The cells of the epidermis originate from the deepest layer of the epidermis, the *stratum basale*, or the basal layer. The cells in this layer, known as the *basal cells*, are the mother cells of most of the cells in the epidermis. New cells are formed in the basal layer and migrate up through the epidermis, taking on different shapes and forming different epidermal layers along the way. These migrating cells reach the end of their journey at the top layer of the epidermis, where they turn into flat, tightly packed discs, called *corneocytes*, and die off. It is this layer of dead skin cells that form the visible layer of the skin and its tough, protective coating, the stratum corneum. Through washing and friction, this layer of dead cells is continually worn off—a process known as *desquamation*—and replaced with a new layer of corneocytes in a cycle of continuous renewal.

The rate at which this cell renewal occurs is important, because it contributes greatly to the appearance of your skin. When you are young, epidermal cells turn over about every thirty days. As you get older, the activity of the cells in the basal layer slows, and they divide more and more slowly. By age eighty, cell turnover takes twice as long as when we were thirty. As a result, the epidermis becomes thinner and more fragile. In addition, the dead skin cells in the top layer of the stratum corneum slough off more slowly, causing the complexion to become dull and lose its glow.

The good news is that the renewal rate of the top layer of the epidermis is affected by how quickly the outer layer of dead cells peels off. When the corneocytes are lost quickly, the cells of the stratum corneum are replaced at a much faster rate. This is the secret behind exfoliation. Exfoliating treatments using alpha hydroxy (AHAs) and beta hydroxy acids (BHAs) increase the rate at which the dead cells in the stratum corneum are peeled off and, as a consequence, speed up renewal of the outer cell layer. As new skin is brought to the surface more rapidly, the skin becomes clearer, more transparent, and fresher looking. Chapter 8 discusses all you need to know about the benefits of exfoliating treatments, how to evaluate exfoliating products, and how and when to use exfoliating techniques as part of a complete anti-aging skin care regimen.

Decreased Nutritional Supply. As we saw above, the epidermis is nourished by innumerable tiny blood vessels in the dermis, which bring a constant flow of vitamins, antioxidants, and other nutrients to the epidermis. In addition, dermal lymph vessels absorb and remove waste products from the cells in the outer layer of the skin.

The junction between the epidermis and the dermis is structured in such a way that the flow of nutrients into the epidermis

is optimized. Instead of simply being a continuous, straight border, the dermal-epidermal juncture is more like a series of rolling
hills between the two layers of skin tissue. This expands the area
of contact between the dermis and the epidermis, magnifying the
flow of nutrients and drainage of waste products.

As we grow older, however, the junction between the epidermis and the dermis grows flatter. As a result, the surface area
between these two skin layers becomes smaller, substantially
reducing blood flow to the epidermis and the effectiveness of
nutrient transfer and waste transportation.

Blood flow to the epidermis helps to give the skin the fresh,
peachy glow of youth. As the nutrient flow to the epidermis
diminishes over time, the complexion becomes increasingly pale
and lifeless, eventually displaying the pasty, sallow hue commonly seen in older people.

Despite the advance of aging, however, there are a number of
things you can do to slow down the rate at which the skin's nutritional supply system declines. Chapters 4 and 5 discuss simple
habits you can adopt to enhance the appearance of your complexion and substantially extend the number of years your skin
radiates a fresh and youthful glow.

Increased Dryness. As we get older, the oil-producing glands in
the dermis enlarge but, paradoxically, excrete less of the skin's
natural moisturizing substance, sebum. As a consequence, the
stratum corneum loses an important component of its protection
against moisture loss and becomes more dry and sensitive.

Increased dryness in the top layer of skin is not just an annoy-
ing cosmetic problem that shows up as fine lines, wrinkles, or
rough, flaky skin; it also impedes the functioning of the skin. The
stratum corneum plays a vital role in protecting the skin from
moisture loss and regulating the rate of evaporation from the skin.
If it becomes too dry, the skin loses some of its ability to retain
water, resulting in increased dryness and initiating a vicious cycle
that causes the protective surface of the skin to break down.

A sufficiently moist environment is also needed for proper functioning of a number of natural enzymes, which play a key role in sloughing off the dead skin cells on the surface of the skin. When the skin is too dry, these enzymes can't do their work effectively, thereby slowing down the process of cell renewal and giving the skin an unhealthy, dull appearance.

A good moisturizer can work wonders for dry, aging skin by restoring the smoothness of parched skin and removing or minimizing the fine lines that result from dry skin. Chapter 7 takes an in-depth look at how moisturizers work, how to evaluate the many different delivery systems used in moisturizers today, and how to choose a moisturizer that is suitable for your skin.

AGE-RELATED CHANGES IN THE DERMIS

Decrease in Dermal Volume. As we age, our dermal mass gradually decreases. The rate of collagen and elastin renewal declines, and the concentration of GAGs becomes lower, reducing the skin's ability to retain water. As the dermal architecture deteriorates, skin starts to lose its plumpness, resilience, and elasticity, and wrinkles begin to proliferate. The effects of gravity gradually become apparent as droopy, sagging skin, particularly on the neck and around the jawline. The wear and tear caused by repeated muscle movements becomes visible as expression lines in the forehead, between the brows, and around the mouth.

The collagen and elastin structures of the dermis deteriorate in a number of ways. The collagen fibers thicken and become less responsive, the collagen bundles become more disorganized, and the effectiveness of collagen repair decreases. The elastin fibers disintegrate as well, becoming fragmented and frayed. As a result, the skin loses resilience and recovers more slowly after stretching.

You can see this change in older skin by doing a "stretch test." In young people, when you pinch a section of skin on the upper part of the hand and let go, it snaps back immediately. In older skin that has lost its elasticity, however, you'll see the so-called tent effect—the skin stays in the shape of a tent for a short while before bouncing back. The older skin gets, the longer it takes to revert to its normal position.

This deterioration in the resilience and elasticity of the skin is a primary factor in the appearance of wrinkles. Although they appear on the surface of the skin, wrinkles are in large part the result of massive deterioration of the supportive structure in the dermis. For this reason, to be effective, cosmetic treatments that seek to slow and reduce the appearance of wrinkles must also address the age-related deterioration of the dermis.

The good news is that in recent years researchers in cosmetic dermatology have developed several ways to slow or even reverse the decline of dermal structures. In women, the majority of the loss of dermal mass happens in the years around menopause, from around forty-five to fifty-five. Chapter 6 surveys different means of slowing these changes. In addition, chapters 9 and 10 introduce new treatments that help to stimulate new collagen production in the dermis, while chapter 11 takes a closer look at the fillers some people use to restore dermal mass mechanically from the outside.

LOSS OF SUBCUTANEOUS TISSUE

The decline in dermal volume is mirrored by a decrease in subcutaneous tissue, the layer of fat that insulates the body and provides a protective cushion beneath the dermis. Unfortunately, this loss of subcutaneous tissue happens selectively—it decreases in the places where we need it, such as the face and hands, and increases in the places where we really don't want excess fat, such as the thighs (in women) and waist (in men).

In the face, the progressive loss of subcutaneous fat may result in indentation in the temple and cheek area, giving a person a

TABLE 2.1

How Your Skin Changes through the Decades

AGE	APPEARANCE	PHYSIOLOGY
Below 15	Nearly perfect skin. Smooth texture, pores small.	Excellent repair capabilities. Low sebaceous gland activity. Skin hydration good.
15–25	Acne key factor in surface texture. Fine lines start to appear, pore size increases.	High sebaceous gland activity (increasing the risk of acne). Mild drop in dermal repair and collagen synthesis. Strong cohesion between skin layers and rapid cell turnover. Small drop in skin hydration, noticed particularly in winter.
25–45	More fine lines and appearance of first wrinkles. Early signs of sagging near the eyes. Some loss of elasticity. Adult acne.	Moderate decrease in dermal repair, resulting in less collagen and increasing accumulation of damaged connective tissue. Noticeable and significant drop in skin hydration.
45–55	More wrinkles, rough texture. Sallow yellow color begins to appear. Pores and age spots enlarge and define. Sagging near eye and cheek.	Significant decrease in dermal repair and continued dermal degradation. Cohesion between skin layers continues to decline. Thinning of epidermis and stratum corneum. Skin tends to be dry.
55+	Wrinkles and fine lines in abundance. Uneven color, pigmentation. Sagging worsens. Dark circles under the eyes.	Compromised dermal repair, abundance of damaged connective tissue. Low production of collagen and sebum.

Gray, 2000, p. 67. Reproduced with permission of Palgrave Macmillan.

somewhat gaunt appearance. In the thighs, accumulation of fatty tissue is one of the factors that give rise to cellulite, the dimpled, "bumpy" thighs that become increasingly common in women in their forties.

There is no way you can avoid getting older, but there are numerous ways to delay the signs of aging. By taking control of the external factors that induce aging of the skin, you can prevent time from engraving its marks on your face—and even take years off your appearance. So let's take a closer look at the many options available to you for slowing the progression of aging.

PART II

Prevention: How to Keep Aging in Check

CHAPTER 3

If You Do Nothing Else, Do This: How to Defeat the Leading Cause of Aging

When Katie first came for a consultation, she was concerned about the many fine wrinkles around her eyes and on her forehead. Only in her late twenties, she was clearly aging prematurely. It didn't take more than one glance to establish the reason why: Katie had a deep, bronze tan. At the same time, her blue eyes, fine-pored skin, and blonde hair made it apparent that her skin was very sensitive to the sun.

It took little questioning to find out that Katie had donned a more or less permanent tan since her college years. She was clearly attached to her copper-toned skin, which she felt made her look healthy and attractive. When asked if she were aware that her tan was probably a contributing factor to the premature wrinkles on her face, Katie looked sheepish and mumbled something or other about using sunscreen most of the time.

Katie is not alone. Public health experts and medical professionals have long warned that excessive exposure to the sun not only ages the skin prematurely, but increases the risk of skin cancer as well. Yet, many people still ignore the warnings. Surveys of people on the beach, for example, show that on any given day only half of beachgoers are wearing sunscreen. And only four out of ten people take researchers' advice and use sunscreen all year round. Close to two out of ten people in this country have never even used a sun care product.

Sunlight is, without comparison, the greatest enemy of the skin. If you're at all concerned about keeping your youthful looks and delaying your skin's aging, you have to take precautions to protect it from the sun. There are no ifs or buts about it.

Even if your skin, like Katie's, has already suffered sun damage, there now are numerous ways to treat and reverse sun damage. By using such treatments and protecting herself from the sun in the future, Katie can undo much of the tissue injury her skin has suffered. Without undergoing such treatments, however, Katie might end up like Sylvia, a woman in her early sixties who has lived most of her life on the southern California seaside. Sylvia insists on entertaining visitors in a darkened room with the shades closed, no matter what time of day. Close up, it becomes apparent why. Unlike Katie's face, where the signs of sun damage have just started to emerge, Sylvia's face is a textbook case of what happens when one spends a lifetime in the sun. Her face is a patchwork of wrinkles covered with numerous blotchy brown spots — clearly a case of sun-induced aging run amok.

It can be hard to recognize just how much sun exposure accelerates skin aging, because it takes years for the full extent of the damage to show up. You might spend a lot of time in the sun and still dodge skin cancer, but when it comes to the aging effects of the sun, you're out of luck. Here, the formula is very simple:

Sun Exposure = Skin Damage = Premature Aging to

Even if your skin type is dark, and you don't suffer the same risk of sunburn as lighter skin types, you are still susceptible to sun damage—albeit to a lesser extent. And you don't have to be a sun worshipper to be at risk. For the vast majority of people, skin damage comes not from spending long hours in the sun. Rather, it is the cumulative effect of small doses of sunlight every day.

The Source of Sun Damage:
Ultraviolet Radiation

The sun emits a wide spectrum of rays. What we perceive as sunlight is only the *visible spectrum of light*, which makes up 39 percent of the rays reaching the earth. *Infrared light,* another component of sunlight, constitutes 56 percent of the sun's rays. Infrared radiation is heat waves, and although you can't perceive infrared radiation with your eyes, you experience it as a pleasant sensation of warmth when the sun hits your skin.

Ultraviolet light, or UV radiation, is only about 5 percent of the sunlight that reaches the earth. Yet this small, invisible fraction of sunlight is far more harmful to the skin than any other part of the sun's rays. There are three types of UV rays: UVA, UVB, and UVC. Most UVC rays are absorbed by the earth's atmosphere and never reach the surface of the planet. Mercifully so, because UVC light causes serious damage to the deoxyribonucleic acid (DNA) of cells and is more dangerous than any other type of ultraviolet light. UVA and UVB radiation, however, are still of great concern for humans. They differ in the type and degree of injury they are capable of inflicting and in how deeply they penetrate the layers of the skin (see figure 3.1).

UVB Light. A useful mnemonic for the effects of UVB light is to think "B" for burn. UVB rays penetrate the epidermis and inflict intense damage on the skin. A sunburn is an inflammatory response and a warning cry from your skin that you've stayed

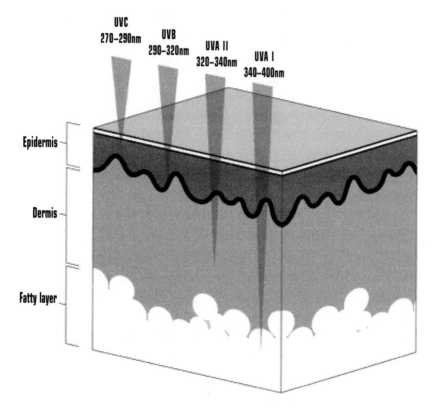

Figure 3.1 The effects of UV rays.

too long in the sun. Although this acute response to UVB radiation is quite unpleasant, it is harmless compared to the long-term effects of UVB light, which include premature aging, weakening of the skin's natural immune protective factors, and substantially increased risk of skin cancer.

UVA Light. To understand the impact of UVA light, think "A" for aging. UVA light permeates even depper into the skin than UVB light, reaching the dermis and parts of the subcutaneous tissue. Although UVA light creates less acute damage than UVB, its long-term effects are just as devastating as those of UVB light, including accelerated aging and heightened skin cancer risk. There are two types of UVA light, long-wave, or UVA-I, and short-wave, or UVA-II. UVA-I is by far more harmful, because it reaches the deepest layers of the skin.

UVA radiation in the atmosphere is about twenty times more plentiful than UVB light. It is not as immediately harmful to the skin as UVB, but it is more constant and insidious. The intensity of UVB light varies greatly with the time of day, season, altitude, weather, and so on. The bombardment of UVA rays, on the other hand, is constant. Unlike UVB light, UVA is not blocked by window glass (think long commutes in the car), and it easily penetrates light clothing. Cloud cover provides some protection against UVB light, while more than 90 percent of UVA light still reaches the earth on a cloudy day.

In other words, you won't develop a sunburn when you go for a walk on a gray winter day, but your skin will still soak up age-accelerating UVA radiation. People who don't spend long hours in the sun often assume that the risks of UV radiation don't apply to them. Unfortunately, that is not true. Researchers estimate that 80 to 90 percent of the UV radiation we receive derives from short, frequent exposures to the head, neck, and hands — when we walk to and from the car, go for a bike ride, exercise outside, and so on. The head, neck, and hands also happen to be the places where premature aging is particularly apparent. In addition, more than 60 percent of the two most common forms of skin cancer occur on these body parts.

How Vulnerable Is Your Skin to the Sun?

The human body has a remarkable ability to adapt to environmental challenges. In regions of the world where the sun is very intense, such as Latin America, India, and the equatorial regions of Africa, the skin of the indigenous people has developed a number of protective mechanisms against sunlight.

The skin contains its own protective sun filter, known as *melanin*, a natural pigment that acts as a shield against the sun's ultraviolet radiation. Melanin granules above the nucleus of a skin cell absorb and reflect UV rays, ward off free radical attacks, and in other ways create a protective shield for the DNA in the vital core of the cell.

The degree of protection you enjoy is determined by the color of your skin, because melanin is also the substance that gives skin its color. In dark skin, melanin production is more plentiful and offers far greater natural protection against sunlight. There are two types of melanin pigment — *eumelanin* granules and *phoemelanin* granules. Eumelanin granules are the most common and offer the best protection. This type of melanin is most abundant in dark or black skin. Pheomelanin granules, on the other hand, are present in higher proportions in people with lighter skin. These granules are lighter and more irregular in shape and do not provide as effective a shield against sunlight as eumelanin.

Highly pigmented dark skin provides about thirty times more pro-

TABLE 3.1   What Is Your Skin Type?

IF YOUR SKIN IS . . .	YOU ARE SKIN TYPE	REACTION TO UV RADIATION
Extremely white and very pale, fine-pored 'porcelain look,' possibly freckled, eyes blue or green.	I	Burns easily and strongly. Doesn't tan.
White and fair with fine pores. Freckles possible.	II	Usually burns, tans slightly and with difficulty.
White to olive, as in peoples of Mediterranean and Mid-European descent.	III	Burns moderately, tans moderately to a golden brown.
Beige or light brown, as in people of Hispanic, darker Mediterranean, Asian, or light Asian-Indian descent.	IV	Burns rarely, tans easily and moderately.
Moderate brown, as in people of African-American, African, dark Asian-Indian, or West Indian descent.	V	Rarely burns; tans to a dark brown.
Dark brown or black as in people of Central African or Australian Aboriginal descent.	VI	Never burns; tans to a deep brown or black.

tection against the sun than fair skin. Black skin also has a thicker epidermis, making it harder for UV rays to penetrate into the dermis. Although dark skin affords greater natural protection, you are still susceptible to UV damage if your skin is type V or VI. (See table 3.1 to determine your skin type.) You may not realize it, however, because type V and VI skin does not turn red when it is burned by the sun. Instead, it gets darker. Although the long-term consequences of sun damage, such as skin cancer and sun-induced aging, are less dramatic among African-Americans and people of Hispanic origin, they do occur.

Characteristics of Sun-Induced Aging

The harmful effects of the sun on the skin are typically referred to as *photodamage*. Similarly, the premature aging induced by the sun is often called *photoaging*. The degree to which photoaging is a factor depends both on skin type and the amount of sun

PHOTOAGING RISK	SKIN CANCER RISK
High. Wrinkles and age spots common around middle age.	Very High
High. Wrinkles and age spots common toward middle age.	Quite high
Moderate to high. Wrinkles somewhat less, brown patches are common.	Moderate
Moderate to low. Tends to develop few wrinkles, brown patches very common.	Low
Low. Wrinkles sparse, but deep; brown patches prevalent.	Low
Low. Very few wrinkles, typically deep.	Very Low

exposure you have received throughout your life. Photoaging is superimposed on and accelerates the normal aging of the skin. It can have a devastating impact on our already fragile aging biological systems, exacerbating the deterioration of skin tissue far beyond what happens during the normal aging process. The impact of photodamage, which is cumulative, shows up in a number of different ways.

As we saw in chapter 2, sunlight increases generation of free radicals, the molecular marauders that snatch electrons from surrounding cells, disrupting the integrity of cellular structures and functions. Free radicals are the medium through which most sun damage is inflicted. The impairment of the cellular environment wrought by free radicals causes the tissue damage associated with photoaging.

The most typical signs of photoaging include:

- *Damaged collagen and elastin fibers.* Collagen fibers deteriorate, and elastin fibers turn into a tangled, amorphous mass of coarse, abnormal fibers, a condition known as *elastosis*. These changes result in premature wrinkles.
- *Decreased hydrating capacity.* The number of glycoproteins in the dermis increases in photodamaged skin, but at the same time, they appear to lose some of their water-binding capacity. Since glycoproteins play a key role in keeping the skin hydrated and supple, this further predisposes the skin to wrinkles. Many researchers believe the changes associated with photodamage are a far more important factor in the appearance of wrinkles than chronological age.
- *Spider veins.* The small blood vessels in the dermis decrease in number and become dilated and malformed, giving rise to a condition known as *telangiectases*, or spider veins. These are also known as "broken" veins and most commonly appear on the nose and cheeks.
- *Age spots.* Prolonged or frequent sun exposure causes skin to permanently increase melanin output. In its more charming

expression, this excess melanin shows up as freckles. However, in older or more sun-damaged skin, these patches of persistent pigmentation show up as unflattering age spots, also known as *solar lentignes.*

•*Dull complexion.* Sun-induced changes in the skin's texture make it appear rougher, lusterless, and more sallow.

Photodamage and Skin Cancer

As unsettling as the exterior signs of photoaging may be, they are just the surface indicators of a more disturbing fact: sun exposure has put you at increased risk of developing skin cancer.

Skin cancer is a factor to be reckoned with. The incidence of skin cancer has taken on almost epidemic proportions in this

A Test for Photoaging

If your skin tone is fair and vulnerable to sunlight, use this simple test to get a sense of how much photodamage you may already have suffered. Take a look at your face and forearms. Now, compare the appearance of these with the skin in an area of your body that has not been exposed to the sun, such as your stomach, breast, or underarms.

In most people who have spent a fair amount of time in the sun, only the skin that has received little sunlight still retains the smooth, soft, and translucent quality of normal, healthy skin. Photodamaged skin, on the other hand, tends to be darker, more coarse, mottled, freckled, uneven, or wrinkled.

country, striking 1.3 million Americans per year and accounting for about half of all new cancer cases every year. One in five Americans will be diagnosed with some form of skin cancer at some point in their lives. The incidence of the most life-threatening form of skin cancer, malignant melanoma, is particularly on the rise; it has increased more than any other cancer in recent years. In 1935, the chance of developing malignant melanoma was one in 1,500. In 1991, it had soared to one in 150, and it is now one in 70.

Sunlight launches a multilevel assault on the skin, which magnifies the risk of developing skin cancer in several ways. First, UV light weakens the skin's normal immune defenses, which constantly monitor the skin for cancerous growths. Second, sunlight causes damage to the DNA of the cells, both directly as radiation and through the production of free radicals, which attack vital cellular structures. Any damage to skin cells' DNA vastly increases a person's risk of contracting skin cancer.

The problem is amplified the older you get, because with age the skin produces less melanin, thus increasing its susceptibility to UV damage. In addition, the DNA's natural ability to repair itself declines as the body ages, impairing one of the body's key defenses against cancer. It is no surprise that the incidence of skin cancer increases dramatically with age.

If skin cancer is caught early, the cure rate is extremely high—up to 95 percent. It does not take expensive medical tests to detect skin cancer. Screen your body once a month, especially if you are a skin type I or II or otherwise fall into a high-risk group. Examine all skin surfaces to see if there are any new moles or growths or changes in existing ones. The most deadly form of cancer, melanoma, often shows up in areas that rarely get sun exposure, so be sure to look under the arms, on the buttocks, on the undersides of the breasts, and in the groin area.

Be particularly watchful for moles that change shape or color, grow larger, or develop an irregular border. If you have a lot of

What Is Your Risk of Developing Skin Cancer?

Take the following quiz to find out whether you fall into a high-, medium-, or low-risk group for developing malignant skin growths.

Your hair color is:
   Blond or red, 4 points; Brunette, 3 points; Black, 2 points
Your eye color is:
   Blue, green, or gray, 4 points; Hazel, 3 points; Brown, black, 2 points
When exposed to the sun for one hour in the summer, you:
   Burn and sometimes blister, 4 points; Burn then tan, 3 points; Tan, 1 point
Do you have freckles?
   Many, 5 points; Some, 3 points; No, 2 points
Occupation Site:
   Outdoors, 4 points; Mixed, 3 points; Indoors, 2 points
Anyone in family had skin cancer?
   Yes, 5 points; No, 1 point
Lived for greatest time prior to age 18 in:
   Southern U.S., 4 points; Midwest U.S., 3 points; Northern U.S., 2 points.

Now, add up the points to see what your risk factor is. If you scored:

26–30 points: Your lifetime risk for skin cancer is very high.

23–25 points: Your lifetime risk for skin cancer is high.

16–22 points: Your lifetime risk for skin cancer is average.

10–15 points: Your lifetime risk for skin cancer is low.

Reprinted with the permission of the American Academy of Dermatology. All rights reserved.

TABLE 3.2   The Three Different Types of Skin Cancer

	CHARACTERISTICS
BASAL CELL CANCER	Small bump or pimple-like nodule; typically round, pink, or skin-colored, pearly surface; may bleed repeatedly.
SQUAMOUS CELL CANCER	Red or pink scaly patch, usually raised. May ulcerate and develop a crust.
MELANOMA	New dark patch, or existing mole changing shape or getting larger. Look for moles with the following features: •Asymmetry •Irregular border •Mixed shades of color •Diameter larger than a pencil eraser •May itch or bleed easily

atypical moles, consider taking a photo of them so your dermatologist has a baseline from which to evaluate whether they are changing shape. You also want to watch out for *actinic keratoses*, skin growths that look like red, warty spots and have a coarse, more sandpaperlike texture than the surrounding skin. These are precancerous growths, which could turn into squamous cell cancer if not removed.

If you notice a suspicious-looking new growth or changes to existing moles or bumps, make an appointment immediately to see a dermatologist. In addition, be sure to get a full-body skin exam by a dermatologist at least once a year.

A number of benign growths may appear on the skin as a result of sun damage, so don't panic if you find a new mole or bump. However, if your skin is light, if you have spent a lot of time in

TYPICAL LOCATIONS	PROGNOSIS
Mostly in sun-exposed areas, such as face, neck, and other sun-exposed areas.	At least 95 percent of incidents curable when discovered early.
Mostly in sun-exposed areas, such as the back of the hands, the edge of the lips, ears, face.	Cure rate high when discovered early.
All over the body, not just in sun-exposed areas. Most common locations: • Women: back, legs • Men: back, chest, abdomen	When caught early, curable in most cases.

the sun, and/or if you have suffered severe sunburns from time to time, stay vigilant and consult with a specialist if you have any doubts. This is what Lillian did, and it saved her life. When she first noticed a new mole in the area around her eyes, she asked her family doctor to take a look at it. He shrugged it off, saying it was a benign growth and nothing to worry about. Lillian kept a close eye on the mole, however, and when she noticed it changing shape, she made an appointment with a dermatologist.

Although the mole was small and looked completely innocuous, the fact that it had changed size raised a red flag for the dermatologist. And sure enough, the mole tested positive as a malignant skin growth. Thanks to Lilian's watchfulness, the cancer was caught very early and could be treated simply by removing the growth and some of the skin around it.

Health Benefits of Sunlight

While excessive sun exposure is a major risk factor for skin cancer, sunlight also confers numerous health benefits. The sun triggers production of vitamin D, which is necessary for calcium absorption and enhances the health of bones, muscles, and the immune system. Vitamin D is also thought to protect against certain cancers, hypertension, and autoimmune diseases. Ten minutes of sun exposure a day will give you all the vitamin D you need.

Sun protection is not just something to do when the need for it is obvious, such as when you're heading off for a day at the beach. Shielding your skin from the sun should be part of your daily routine, like brushing your teeth or putting on moisturizer. Photodamage starts within minutes after you step out into the sun. If your skin is continuously exposed to small doses of UV radiation because it's not adequately protected, the aging slide will continue unabated. As we have seen, up to 80 percent of skin's aging is due to sun exposure, so take all the steps you can to shield your skin from the sun. It is the best wrinkle prevention you can ever get.

The Pros and Cons of Sunscreens

Regular use of sunscreens not only protects you against sunburn and skin cancer, but from premature aging of the skin as well. However, sunscreens do have limitations. You need to be aware of these to know how to benefit from sunscreen use and how to take additional steps to shield your skin from the sun.

Skin Cancer Rates and the Thinning Ozone Layer

The incidence of skin cancer has been steadily on the rise in Western societies, at a rate of 4 percent per year. Most researchers agree that the incidence of skin cancer has increased because people spend more time in the sun. However, an increasing number of scientists are also voicing concerns about another potential risk factor—the thinning of the ozone layer.

The ozone layer shields us from the sun's harmful radiation by absorbing much of the radiation from the sun, particularly UVB and UVC light, and preventing it from reaching the surface of the earth. However, there is mounting scientific evidence that the ozone layer is being depleted due to the effects of pollutants released into the earth's atmosphere.

Depletion of the ozone layer has been calculated at 3 to 9 percent in North America and other temperate zones. Researchers have predicted that with each 1 percent decrease in ozone level, the incidence and mortality from skin cancer will increase correspondingly. The Environmental Protection Agency has forecast a 1 to 2 percent increase in melanoma mortality alone with each 1 percent decrease in ozone. For this reason, it is more important than ever to protect yourself adequately from the sun when you are outside.

When sunscreens were first developed, UVB radiation was assumed to be the main cause of sunburn, photoaging, and skin cancer. As a consequence, the first sunscreens were formulated to shield the skin from UVB rays only. Although UVA rays now are thought to be more potent cancer-causing agents than UVB rays, this determination is fairly recent, and sunscreen manufacturers

The Informed Consumer

THE MIRAGE OF THE SAFE TAN

Although UVA light is no longer considered safe for the skin, it is the main type of UV-radiation used in the still widely popular tanning beds. The aging effects of UVA damage do not show up for years, but when they do, they can be hard to reverse. If having a tanned look is important to you, do your skin—and yourself—a favor and use one of the many excellent self-tanning creams now available. They are the only safe way to get a tanned appearance.

The secret to using tanning creams is to apply them to a smooth and even surface. Follow these steps to get the best results:

- *Exfoliate lightly.* Exfoliate the skin gently by applying a scrubbing cleanser or an AHA or BHA product (see chapter 8), or by rubbing the skin lightly with a wet washcloth.
- *Shower.* Take a quick shower and towel dry. Don't use soap, as this may leave a thin film of alkaline residue on the skin that interferes with the active agent of the tanning cream.
- *Apply.* Apply a thin, even layer of the self-tanner to the areas you

(continued on next page)

are still playing catch-up. As a consequence, only some of the sunscreens on the market today provide adequate protection against both UVA and UVB radiation.

HOW TO EVALUATE THE EFFECTIVENESS OF A SUNSCREEN

The sun protection factor (SPF) of a sunscreen provides a somewhat crude measure of its protective value. It tells you how long the product allows you to stay in the sun without developing a

THE INFORMED CONSUMER (*continued*)

want to have a tanned look. It's better to apply too little than too much; you can always apply more later. Divide the body into sections and cover one section at a time before you move on to the next. Start with your face, taking care to avoid the hairline, and continue with your neck and shoulders.

• *Vary your application.* Areas with thicker skin, such as the elbows and knees, absorb more color, so apply a very thin layer of tanning cream in these areas. Be particularly careful with skin areas where there are creases, such as the neck, and dab off any excess cream with a tissue.

• *Wash your hands.* To avoid darkening of your palms and nails, wash your hands thoroughly immediately after application.

• *Allow enough time to dry.* Allow at least twenty minutes before getting dressed. Remember that it takes eight to twenty-four hours for the full darkening effect to develop.

• *Reapply.* To maintain the color, reapply the self-tanner every two to four days. The face requires more frequent reapplication.

Never apply a tanning cream without first trying a small test patch, for example, on the underside of the arm. Then wait until the next day to see if the color suits you and to make sure you don't develop an allergic reaction.

sunburn. Let's say, for example, that your skin gets red from UVB radiation after you spend ten minutes in bright sunlight without any form of protection. If you apply a lotion with an SPF 15, the time you can spend in the sun before developing a sunburn is multiplied by 15. So you can now stay in the sun for 150 minutes, or two and a half hours, without developing redness. Similarly, a sunscreen with SPF 30 would allow you to stay in the sun 10 minutes x 30 = 300 minutes, or five hours, before your skin turns red.

TABLE 3.3
FDA-Approved Sunscreen Ingredients and Their Allowed Concentration

UVA-I/UVA-II	UVA-II/UVB	UVB
Avobenzone (Parsol 1789) (2–3%)	Oxybenzone (6%)	Aminobenzoic acid (15%)
Zinc oxide* (20%)	Dioxybenzone (3%)	Cinoxate (3%)
Titanium oxide* (25%)	Sulisobenzone (10%)	Homosalate (15%)
	Meradimate (5%)	Octocrylene (10%)
		Octinoxate (7.5%)
		Octisalate (5%)
		Padimate O (8%)
		Ensulizole (4%)
		Trolamine salicylate (12%)

*Zinc oxide and titanium oxide also afford UVB protection.

The problem is that the redness of a sunburn is a very incomplete measure of the degree of damage your skin suffers. First, the skin sustains photodamage long before visible signs of sunburn can be detected. Second, since a sunburn is induced mostly by UVB rays, the SPF tells you nothing about the extent to which the product protects against the age-accelerating, cancer-inducing effects of UVA light.

The U.S. Food and Drug Administration (FDA) is developing new guidelines for how manufacturers must label a product's UVA-protective factor. Currently, a company may claim that its sunscreen offers broad-spectrum UVA/UVB protection simply by including one ingredient that filters UVA light, but it may not cover the entire spectrum of UVA light.

One way to gauge the effectiveness of a sunscreen is to look at the ingredient list. As you will recall, UVA light is divided into long-wave light, or UVA-I, and short-wave light, or UVA-II. Most UVB-protective ingredients also offer protection against UVA-II light.

The Informed Consumer

HOW TO DETERMINE THE EFFECTIVENESS
OF A SUNSCREEN PRODUCT
Your best bet for finding a safe and effective sunscreen
product is to look for those with the Skin Cancer
Foundation's Seal of Recommendation on the label. Such products
satisfy stringent criteria for effectiveness. They must have an SPF of
15 or greater, and the SPF must have been validated by testing on
twenty people. In addition, test results must be within acceptable
limits for phototoxic reactions and contact irritation. Any claims
that the sunscreen is water- or sweat-resistant must also be substantiated by the manufacturer. Sunglasses and other protective
products, such as window glass film and sun-protective clothing,
can be granted the seal as well.

For a list of sunscreens and other products carrying the
seal, go to the Skin Care Foundation's website at
www.skincancer.org/aboutus/seal.html.

However, only three ingredients approved for use in the United
States protect against long-wave UVA-I, the most harmful type of
UVA light, which causes damage at the deepest layers of the skin.

When you buy a sunscreen, look for products that contain at
least one of the three ingredients that filter UVA-I light: avobenzone (Parsol 1789), zinc oxide, or titanium oxide. (Mexoryl SX is
another effective UVA-I filtering ingredient, but it is only
approved for use outside the United States.) Avobenzone is a
chemical agent that absorbs UV radiation, and zinc oxide and
titanium oxide are physical agents that stay on the surface of the
skin and reflect ultraviolet radiation. Studies have shown that
sunscreens containing avobenzone tend to be the most effective,

Ask the Doctor

Q. *I've heard that sunscreens don't even afford the protection against UVB radiation and sunburn that the SPF indicates. Is that true?*

A. Yes and no. The SPF reflects the laboratory value of a sunscreen's protective factor; however, the effectiveness of a sunscreen is diminished if it is not used properly. Researchers estimate that the typical sunscreen user only gets 20 to 50 percent of the SPF protection indicated, because the sunscreen is applied too thinly or unevenly. The SPF value is based on applying a coating of about an ounce to the entire body and half to one teaspoon to the face. In addition, sunscreen wears off when we perspire, go swimming, or our skin rubs against our clothes.

One way to get around this problem is to use a sunscreen with a higher SPF, so that even if you apply the product too thinly, you're still likely to get at least an SPF 15. Unfortunately, products with higher SPFs contain a higher concentration of active ingredients and are more likely to cause irritation or allergic reactions in people with sensitive skin.

Another approach is to apply the sunscreen twice. Put on a coating fifteen to thirty minutes before you go out to give the protective film adequate time to soak into the skin. Then follow up with another application fifteen to thirty minutes after going out in the sun. This not only results in a thicker layer of protective sunscreen, it is also likely to cover spots you might have missed the first time around.

If you go swimming, use a product that is water-resistant. Many standard sunscreens will wash off after twenty minutes in the water. In addition, if you spend a long time in the sun, reapply your sunscreen after two to three hours because some protective ingredients break down in sunlight.

particularly when they also contain titanium dioxide. (FDA regulations forbid the combination of avobenzone and zinc oxide.) This effect is completely unrelated to a product's SPF value.

OTHER WAYS TO SHIELD YOUR SKIN FROM UV RADIATION

Sunscreen use alone is not enough to protect your skin against the damaging effects of the sun. You need to take additional measures to avoid premature aging of the skin and increased risk of skin cancer. You can do your skin and yourself a great favor by observing a few simple guidelines:

- *Cut back.* Avoid spending extended periods of time in the sun between 10 A.M. and 4 P.M., when UV radiation is at its strongest. UV light is also more intense in the summer and at high altitudes. For more information on the degree of UV radiation in your area, look for the Ultraviolet Index (UVI), which is featured in many local newspapers and radio stations or on television. You can also find it at the Environmental Protection Agency's website, at www.epa.gov/sunwise/uvindex.html. The UVI index measures the amount of UV radiation reaching your area at noon on a scale from zero (lightest exposure) to ten (most intense exposure).
- *Cover up.* Clothing affords the best means of sun protection. The fabric should be tightly woven, and darker colors provide better protection. Wear a wide-brimmed hat with a tight weave to shield your face from sunlight. A baseball cap does not provide sufficient shade.
- *Watch out on cloudy days.* When you don't feel the warmth of the sun on your skin, you might assume that you're not being exposed to sunlight. Wrong! Clouds block only part of the sun's light spectrum, mainly the infrared rays that produce the sensation of warmth on our skin. A moderate cloud cover

Beauty Secrets of the Rich and Famous

Ever wonder how actress Nicole Kidman has managed to keep her delicate ivory skin smooth and perfect? Kidman's lovely complexion is particularly noteworthy since she grew up in Australia, where the sun's intensity is notorious for accelerating skin aging and skin cancer rates.

To protect her skin while she was growing up, Kidman opted out of spending weekends on the beach with her school friends. Instead, she looked for other fun-filled weekend activities that she could do out of the sun. She found the perfect solution—taking acting classes in a local downtown theater. Thus began Kidman's journey toward her successful acting career.

Although there is no need to avoid outdoor activities altogether, the rest of us would do well to take a lesson from Kidman and develop weekend activities that don't involve spending a lot of time in direct sun.

blocks as little as 10 percent of UVB light. You need to take just as many precautions to protect your skin on cloudy days as on sunny ones.

- *Shade isn't enough.* Sunlight is reflected off any light surface, be it sand, snow, or even concrete. If you sit under an awning or sun umbrella, 50–85 percent of the sun's reflected rays may still hit you.
- *Consider using a window filter.* Glass blocks UVB, but not UVA rays. If your skin is very sensitive to the sun, or if you spend a considerable time commuting in a car every day, consider getting a protective coating for your home and/or car. Several

commercial products are now available that block UV radiation but still allow visible light to shine through. Look for such products as Llumar UV Shield™ or Vista® Window film by CPFilms, Inc.

• *Use antioxidant protection.* The skin uses antioxidants to neutralize excess free radicals generated by sunlight. These antioxidants include vitamin C, vitamin E, beta carotene, and coenzyme Q10. With extended exposure to sunlight, the amount of these antioxidants in the skin is depleted and must be replenished. Vitamin C can be applied topically with good results. The most-researched vitamin C creams are those that contain the L-ascorbic acid type of vitamin C. In addition, researchers recommend taking a combination of antioxidants orally, such as vitamins C and E, to increase the skin's antioxidant reserves.

• *Don't forget the eyes.* UVB radiation contributes to several different forms of eye damage, including cataracts, which affect millions of Americans every year. To avoid harm to your eyes, wear sunglasses whenever you spend time in bright sunlight. Not all sunglasses block UV radiation, so you need to look for ones with a label that specifies UV blocking. Also, be sure to wear sunglasses that wrap around the eyes. Sunlight that reaches the eyes from the sides is particularly harmful, because pupils are dilated behind sunglasses.

Taking steps to prevent sun damage is without a doubt the most powerful anti-aging strategy you can adopt. If your skin has already suffered photodamage, you also might want to consider undergoing some of the important photorejuvenating treatments that have emerged within recent years. These are described in greater detail in chapters 9 and 10. On the prevention side, you can use a number of additional potent approaches to prolong and even restore your youthful looks. We turn to these in the following chapters.

CHAPTER 4

Yes You Can! How to Slow the Aging Clock

*O*n October 29, 1998, seventy-seven-year-old astronaut John Glenn blasted into orbit for the second time in his life. The event marked a personal victory for Glenn, who became the oldest astronaut ever to fly into space. The launch also made medical history. Space travel is one of the most challenging tasks a person can take on, and Glenn's mission was no exception. In nine days, his *Discovery* spacecraft circled the earth 134 times, covering 3.6 million miles in about 213 hours. For the average seventy-seven-year-old, even a sixteen-hour flight halfway around the globe would be a daunting undertaking.

How could Glenn tackle a task that most men half his age would have been incapable of? In the answer to this question lies one of the greatest beauty secrets you will ever find.

Aging is a highly relative phenomenon; it does not unfold according to a fixed, immutable timetable. When measured in years, we all age at the same rate. When measured in terms of the decline of bodily functions, however, aging progresses at a widely different pace from person to person. It is not uncommon to find people well into their fifties who still maintain the youthful vitality and appearance of someone in their late thirties. Conversely, some people appear to have gotten "old before their time," looking overdue for cosmetic surgery by their late thirties.

To explain the difference in the way aging unfolds from person to person, some scientists make a distinction between a person's *chronological age* and his or her *biological age*. Your chronological age is your age in years. Your biological age, on the other hand, is a measure of the degree of wear and tear on your body as indicated by the functional integrity of different organs and bodily systems. Some researchers contend that this biological age is a more important and reliable indicator of a person's potential life span and risk of developing chronic disease.

How is a person's biological age measured? Researchers have proposed a number of physiological measurements, or *biomarkers,* that indicate the health of specific organs and organ systems and the body as a whole. The distinction between chronological and biological age was introduced by Dr. Irwin Rosenberg and his colleagues at Tufts University's Human Nutrition Research Center. Rosenberg proposed numerous biomarkers to measure a person's biological age, including aerobic capacity, blood sugar tolerance, lean muscle mass, reduced basal metabolic rate, ratio of body fat to muscle, cholesterol/high-density lipoprotein (HDL) ratio, blood pressure, bone density, and internal temperature regulation.

You might have noticed that several of the biomarkers listed above also predict a person's risk of developing chronic disease. Blood pressure and cholesterol/HDL ratio, for example, are well-known measures of the heart's health, and blood sugar tolerance indicates a person's risk of contracting diabetes. An abnormal reading on one or several of these biomarkers can be seen as an early warning of premature aging and/or chronic disease.

Spotlight on Research

ARE WRINKLES A BIOMARKER FOR AGING?
Are wrinkles an indicator of a person's general
health status and biological age? Some researchers
think so. M. B. Purba et al. (2001), studied a group of
elderly people by measuring the amount of wrinkling in areas of
their skin that had not been exposed to the sun. They then compared the degree of wrinkling with the subjects' general health status, lifestyle habits, and overall well-being.

People in poor general health and people with poor lifestyle
habits tended to have a higher degree of skin wrinkling. In contrast,
people with the lowest degree of wrinkling enjoyed enhanced
immunity; decreased risk of heart disease, osteoporosis, and cancer;
higher energy levels; clearer thinking; and increased well-being.
This group also had the highest levels of dehydroepiandrosterone
(DHEA), a "youth hormone" associated with slower aging. The
researchers concluded that people with a younger biological age
display less skin wrinkling, independent of their chronological age.

Glenn was able to undertake his mission into space because his
body's biomarkers retained values equivalent to those of a
healthy, much younger man. All his organ systems were func-
tionally intact.

What causes differences between a person's chronological and
biological age to occur? Genetics play a role. Some people are
lucky enough to be born into families whose members tend to
live a long time. But many other factors have equal, if not greater,
impact. Remember the concept of extrinsic skin aging discussed
in chapter 1? Extrinsic aging is caused by environmental factors
that tax the skin—and the body as a whole—such as cigarette

smoke, environmental toxins, air pollutants, and so on. Extrinsic aging is also affected by lifestyle habits, such as the food we eat, the amount of exercise we get, the level of stress we experience in our daily life, and how much sleep we get at night. Over the course of a lifetime, these factors exert considerable impact on our health and physical appearance. It is sometimes said that until the age of forty, we have the face we got from our parents. After forty, we have the face we deserve. Over time, the effects of a lifestyle filled with stress, inadequate nutrition, or too little sleep will be indelibly etched onto the face and skin. Likewise, a healthy lifestyle can do much to slow the advance of time and preserve a youthful appearance.

Some researchers contend that healthy lifestyle habits are the closest we will ever come to a magic bullet — that is, a universal remedy that can effectively treat a host of mental, emotional, and physical ailments. Pick any health problem commonly associated with age. With few exceptions, healthy lifestyle habits will have a positive impact on it. Even genetic heritage can be modified by lifestyle factors. A person who has a family history of diabetes, for example, can reduce the likelihood of ever developing the disease by adopting dietary habits that keep the body's glucose metabolism in balance. Similarly, a person with a genetic predisposition toward heart disease can beat the odds by keeping in shape, keeping blood cholesterol levels low, and so on.

In short, the difference between our age in years and our bodily age arises in large part from factors entirely within our control. Dr. Michael Roizen, a professor at the University of Chicago Hospitals and author of the book *Real Age — Are You as Young as You Can Be?*, analyzed the mortality rates in more than twenty-five thousand medical studies and concluded that our behaviors affect how the aging process unfolds in numerous ways. Dr. Roizen estimates that the simple act of adopting more healthy habits could make it possible to reduce one's biological age by as much as twenty years.

How Well Are You Aging?

The list below will give you a sense of how well you are aging compared to the average woman in your age group. Look at the table and identify any age markers you already have. Then compare the age at which they appeared to the average age at which these markers emerge for other women. This will give you an idea of the rate at which your biological aging is unfolding compared to the average.

AGE MARKER	AGE WHEN 50% OF WOMEN HAVE HAD THIS MARKER DEVELOP	AGE WHEN 75% OF WOMEN HAVE HAD THIS MARKER DEVELOP
Circles under eyes	40	50
Wrinkles on brow	42	52
Intereyebrow wrinkles	44	53
Wrinkles under eyes	46	53
Bags under eyes	47	56
Crow's-feet	49	56
Age spots	52	59
Fine lines on lips	52	59
Wrinkles around lips	55	59
Wrinkled neck	57	60
Wrinkled face	58	61

The table lists the typical signs of aging (column one), the age by which 50 percent of women will exhibit these (column two), and the age by which 75 percent of women have developed this age marker (column three). Take the example of wrinkles on the brow. In a typical group of women, half of them will develop this marker by age forty-two. By age fifty-two, three out of four, or 75 percent, will exhibit this age marker. That is a considerable difference!

SOURCE: CE.R.I.E.S. (CEntre de Recherches et d'Investigations Epidermiques et Sensorielles) of Chanel, 1998.

The three major lifestyle factors that influence your appearance over the long term are the food you eat, the amount of exercise you get, and how much stress you are exposed to. Improving your health habits in just one of these areas can slow down the rate at which your body decays over time. Taking up health routines that address all three areas can literally make you feel — and look — like a million dollars!

In this and the following chapter, we show you how to use your daily habits to take control of the aging process and slow down the relentless ticktock of the clock. We first focus on exercise and stress management. Diet is such a vital component of skin health and overall health that it deserves a chapter of its own and is covered in chapter 5.

Exercising for Health and Beauty

Pick any health problem commonly associated with age — exercise will likely reverse or, at the very least, improve it. Regular moderate exercise is an unfailing strategy for preserving health and slowing down the decay of your body and your appearance. Indeed, some researchers argue that exercise and diet should be considered as medical treatments, because both can relieve a host of mental, emotional, and physical ailments.

Exercise cuts the risk of the leading killer diseases, such as heart disease, cancer, and stroke, and it protects against many of the dreaded diseases of aging, including diabetes, osteoporosis, and arthritis. It also reverses several biomarkers of biological age. It builds aerobic capacity, for example, a measure of the muscles' ability to absorb oxygen for use as fuel, which otherwise declines by an average of 9 percent per decade after age thirty. Researchers have found that there is a direct relationship between how fit a person is (as indicated by a treadmill test) and his or her life expectancy.

When it comes to the skin, exercise is a tonic for youth. It firms the skin by enhancing muscle tone, which in turn smoothes the skin. It also does wonders for your skin tone, because it stimulates blood flow and capillary development, bringing more vital nutrients to the cells and increasing the skin's overall vitality. Take a look at yourself in the mirror after forty-five minutes of vigorous exercise, and you will see the healthy, radiant glow of your youth partly returned. People in poor physical condition, in contrast, inevitably develop flabby and pasty-looking skin.

If all of this is not enough to get you off the couch, consider the effects of exercise on your mental and emotional well-being. Vigorous physical activity stimulates the release of mood-enhancing endorphins and reduces the levels of the stress hormone, cortisol. The result is improved mood and increased happiness, energy, and zest for life. Exercise is one of the most effective nonmedicinal ways of relieving anxiety and preventing or treating mild to moderate depression. And, of course, when you are happier and feel better about yourself, you are naturally more attractive.

A PIECE OF CAKE—OR A WALK IN THE PARK?

You need not launch a training program suitable for the Olympics to reap the benefits of exercise. Something as simple as a daily brisk thirty-minute walk will do the trick. Walking produces many of the health benefits that more intense forms of exercise, such as aerobics and jogging, provide. By some estimates, if all Americans engaged in simple regular exercise, such as walking, thirty minutes a day, it would cut the incidence of chronic diseases in this country by 30 to 40 percent! Walking is also one of the safest ways to exercise; it doesn't put as much pressure on the knees as jogging, and the risk of injury is minimal.

Weight lifting—or strength and resistance training as it is also called—is another type of exercise where even modest efforts pay

Ask the Doctor

A PANACEA FOR CELLULITE?

Q. *I've tried numerous treatments for cellulite on my thighs and buttocks, but I am really disappointed with the results. Someone suggested I try exercise. Would that make a difference?*

A. Cellulite is one of the most dreaded signs of aging. It is unflattering and, unfortunately, hard to treat. Cellulite emerges when the fat layers in the thighs, hips, and buttocks expand. Because of the way the skin is structured, this does not happen evenly, but rather produces the dimpled, bulging look of cellulite.

There is no shortage of creams, lotions, and exotic treatments purporting to remove or alleviate cellulite, but precious little research has demonstrated any consistent effects of these treatments (for more on these, see chapter 12). Exercise is one of the most effective ways of preventing or reducing cellulite.

Strengthening the muscles makes the skin more taut and smooth, thereby reducing the dimpling of cellulite. It is easiest to prevent cellulite by establishing a regular exercise routine early on. However, even if you already have developed cellulite, exercise will trim the extra padding around your hips and thighs and tone and firm your skin. Best of all, it is free (or comes at the cost of a health club membership), and it confers a plethora of additional benefits for your well-being and appearance.

off big-time. Weight training prevents loss of muscle mass, a cause of numerous age-related ills. Strong muscles produce stronger bones, thus preventing osteoporosis. In addition, the energy needs of well-developed muscles cause your body to burn excess calories, keeping you slimmer and protecting you against the health threats commonly associated with overweight.

TABLE 4.2

Fitness Strategies

HEALTHY ADVICE FROM EXERCISE SPECIALISTS

Decide which of the following fitness levels best characterizes you, then choose the exercise strategies that go with it. (Always consult with your doctor before starting any exercise program.)

EXERCISE LEVEL 1   GETTING STARTED

Choose This Level If

- You have never excerised regularly

- You haven't exercised regularly for a while

- You are overweight

How Much Time to Spend

When you're just starting out, 20 minutes of exercise a day, 6 days a week is enough to build your fitness and strength.

If time is an issue, don't do it all in one chunk. Rather, accumulate the 20 minutes during the day by increasing your level of physical activity. Make a game of collecting exercise points, one for each minute you increase your physical activity.

Many people find walking to be the easiest and most enjoyable exercise when they are just starting out. To get health benefits, walk briskly enough to speed up your heart rate and break a light sweat.

Ways to Get Going

- Park a couple of blocks from your work and walk the rest of the way. Or, when shopping, pick the parking spot farthest away from the entrance. (Bonus: You won't have to spend time look for a parking spot.)

- Use the stairs instead of the escalator in the mall or the elevator at work. If you work on the fifth floor, ride to the third floor and take the stairs the rest of the way.

- Instead of keeping up with your friends from the comfort of your couch, grab your cell phone and go for a walk and talk.

- Buy a couple of weights. Bring them on your walks or watch TV and pump iron.

- Just for the fun of it, try a pedometer. This $15 gadget clips to your belt and keeps track of how many steps you walk a day. Aim to build gradually to 10,000 steps, or accumulate about 70,000 steps per week. (It's not as hard as it may seem—even couch potatoes log 2,000 to 4,000 steps a day.

When to Move On

If you are new to exercise, stay on this level for 6 weeks. By then you should be ready to move on to Level 2.

(Continued on next page)

TABLE 4.2—Continued

EXERCISE LEVEL 2   MAINTAIN AND ADVANCE YOUR FITNESS LEVEL

Choose This Level If
- You are already exercising regularly or you have been at Exercise Level 1 for at least 6 weeks.

How Much Time to Spend
Once you have graduated from Level 1, your stronger physical condition will help overcome much of the inertia and lack of energy that otherwise can be a barrier to physical activity. Gradually work up to 30 minutes of physical activity a day, 6 days a week. Alternatively, you can exercise 60 minutes, 3 days a week.

Ways to Get Going
- Have fun. The key to expanding your fitness at this stage is to find physical activities you really enjoy. Explore different activities and see what works for you: jazz dance, ballroom dancing, weight training, membership in a health club, a brisk walk outdoors with a friend, a video workout at home, a team sport, and so on.
- Once you find something you like, enroll in a structured exercise program two to three times a week.
- When possible, exercise early in the day. Then you won't have to think about how to fit in exercise the rest of the day, and you will have all day to enjoy the feeling of accomplishment.
- Get a buddy. Having to be somewhere at a specific time because you made a commitment to a friend is the best way to avoid those last-minute excuses.
- Alternatively, make exercise appointments for yourself. Enter time for exercise sessions in your day timer, calendar, or whatever you use to keep track of appointments.

When to Move On
If you find yourself wanting to charge ahead to Exercise Level 3 after 6 weeks, congratulations! Many people find that the increased feeling of energy, strength, and well-being that comes with growing fitness becomes its own motivation for surging forward.

(Continued on next page)

The key to building fitness is to begin slowly and build up gradually. The body needs time to build muscle mass and expand aerobic capacity, and you need time to make exercise a natural part of your daily routine. If you launch an exercise routine that is too ambitious, you are more likely to get discouraged and give up.

TABLE 4.2—Continued

EXERCISE LEVEL 3

Choose This Level If

- You have followed Exercise Level 2 for at least 6 weeks or you are already in good shape.

How Much Time to Spend

35–45 minutes of physical activity a day will continue to increase your fitness and keep you at a maximum level of health and strength. At this level, pay close attention to the basics of exercise. Spend time warming up and cooling down and stretching. Make sure you drink enough water to replenish fluids lost during your workout. Drink an 8-ounce glass of water before and after your workout and sip water throughout.

Ways to Get Going

- Continue what you have been doing, it obviously works for you. Look for ways to increase the amount of time you spend exercising every day.

- If you particularly enjoy a specific form of exercise, work on perfecting your skills in that area. The mental challenge will add fun to your workout and enhance your sense of accomplishment.

- If no one type of exercise hooks you, develop a repetoire of different activities you enjoy and change them frequently.

- Keep at it. Staying fit is an ongoing project. No matter how fit you are, you could lose up to 90 percent of your fitness in just 3 months if you cut your exercise routine from 5 days a week to 1 day a week.

- Remember to take a day of rest every week; your body needs time to recharge.

From Distressing to De-stressing

Deadlines. Packed schedules. Too little time. Too little money. Too many demands. Too little energy.

As the pace of life grows ever more frantic, symptoms of stress and stress-related disorders are becoming increasingly common.

Stress affects our health and well-being in more ways than most of us realize. Stomach complaints, headaches, and muscle tension are the most familiar short-term effects of stress. Long-term effects include high blood pressure, suppression of the immune system, depression, and anxiety. Stress is also thought to play a role in the development of heart disease and stroke.

Hormonal changes associated with stress are known to cause numerous skin problems, such as acne, thinning of the skin, and itching, or skin disorders such as psoriasis, hives, or shingles. But stress undermines the health of the skin in many subtle ways as well. Stress is a considerable factor in the premature aging of the skin. When the body is under stress, nutrients are redirected from the skin to the vital organs, such as the heart, brain, and lungs. Over time, this deprives the skin of the nourishment it needs for its functioning. Extended periods of stress also affect metabolic functions, slowing down the renewal of skin cells and causing the skin to look dull and gray. Furthermore, stress upsets the body's fluid balance, dehydrating the skin and causing it to sag.

Psychological stress also disrupts the skin's barrier function — the thin oily barrier that seals in moisture and shields the skin from environmental assaults. Once the skin barrier is compromised, the skin becomes excessively dry, more prone to wrinkles, and vulnerable to harmful outside substances. Stress may also induce subclinical inflammation in the skin, unleashing a cascade of molecular changes that causes cumulative tissue damage and accelerates skin aging. As if this weren't enough, stress greatly contributes to extrinsic aging by unleashing a well-known foe — free radicals. It greatly increases oxidative damage to vital cellular structures and functions of the skin and other bodily organs.

STRATEGIES FOR DEFEATING STRESS

Cutting back on stress is one of the most important investments you can make in your long-term health. Anything you do to reduce stress will enhance your appearance and slow down the rate of wear and tear on your body.

You won't be able to get rid of stress altogether—after all, life happens. Nor is it desirable to do so; when handled right, even stressful challenges can be an important impetus for personal growth and progress. There are two ways to address feelings of stress. You can try to reduce the level of stress in your life or you can increase your ability to cope with stress. In practice, both approaches work hand in hand. Coping skills provide a temporary way to deal with stress, and working to reduce stress gets at the root of the problem and provides long-term improvement.

Psychologists have charted several different types of coping skills that people use to deal with stress: physical, mental, social, and spiritual. Here is a broad selection:

- *Exercise.* Exercise is a great stress buster—it strengthens the body and its ability to adapt to and recover from stress. Exercise also triggers mood-enhancing brain chemicals that relax you, improve your well-being, and clear worries from your mind.
- *Steer clear of crutches.* Sugar, caffeine, junk food, and cigarettes may provide short-term relief from stress. Unfortunately, these unhealthy habits put a strain on your body and reduce its ability to cope with stress.
- *Keep your perspective.* Don't get so hung up on your worries and problems that you no longer see the broader picture. Instead, change your focus. Take off for the weekend, go to a concert, do something fun with your kids. Once you take your mind off your problems, they won't seem so overpowering.
- *Remember to enjoy.* Pause to take a deep breath in the midst of rush hour traffic. Watch the colors of the fading day. Listen to relaxing music. Take the dog for a walk. Spend an hour in the garden. Anything that restores you, lifts your spirits, and makes you feel whole will invite greater peace, serenity, and contentment into your life.

- *Find opportunities to laugh.* Laughter releases tension and purifies your emotions, leaving your feeling more carefree, hopeful, and lighthearted.
- *Spend time with your friends.* Share your feelings, worries, dreams, and anxieties with a close friend, relative, professional counselor, or support group. A strong social network is one of the best defenses against stressful life events.
- *Practice relaxation.* Relaxation techniques soothe the body and mind and combat stress. Schedule time for a calming massage once a week, learn to meditate, take up yoga or another program known to provide deep physical and mental relaxation and release. According to research, regular practice of a meditation technique known as the Transcendental Meditation® program can cut biological aging by fifteen to twenty years!
- *Get enough sleep.* Don't forget this important antistress, anti-aging, antieverything antidote. A good night's sleep heals, soothes, restores, refreshes, and rejuvenates the body and mind. It increases energy and triggers the secretion of growth hormone, which is critical for tissue renewal and repair. Sleep has numerous psychological benefits as well; it improves mood; enhances learning; and increases cognitive abilities, memory, and creativity. Research suggests that people who get enough sleep live longer and enjoy a healthier old age.
- *Cut back on stress.* Take a long look at your life and see what causes you to feel stressed and worn-out. Determine which stressful parts of your life can be changed, then make a long-term plan for change. It might take several years to realize the changes you want to make, but even the act of planning for change will make you feel better.
- *Practice time management.* Get essential tasks out of the way first—even if you don't feel like doing them—and prioritize the rest. Don't try to do too much at once. Keep a list and check off the tasks as you go along. This will chart your progress and give you a sense of accomplishment.

• *Work on your people skills.* If conflicts with family members or co-workers are common sources of frustration or anger, take up the challenge. Look to see how you might be able to improve your people skills. Do you always have to be right, or do you need to learn to give in more often? Can you steer clear of quarrels and simply discuss the situation more soberly when tempers have subsided? Are there ways you tend to react that might set other people off? Are there times when you need to be more understanding and tolerant of other people's needs and viewpoints?

The combination of stress management and regular exercise is a potent formula for increasing well-being, because each builds on the other. Being physically fit endows your body with greater resources to adapt to stress, and the very act of exercising purges mind and body from feelings of anxiety and pressure. Conversely, controlling the level of stress in your life will make it easier for you to stick to an exercise routine and avoid unhealthy habits.

Proper exercise and stress management must be combined with a healthy diet to produce their full anti-aging effects. New discoveries in nutrition have made it clear that our daily intake of food affects our health and appearance dramatically, and that it does so in many more ways than previously realized. In the following chapter, we explore the many exciting avenues through which you can use your daily intake of food to slow the aging process and retain a youthful appearance.

CHAPTER 5

Healthy Eating Means Healthy Skin

*P*ut a well-preserved thirty-five-year-old woman with no wrinkles or lines next to a seventeen-year-old with unblemished skin. What will reveal the difference in their ages?

Ignore for a moment the fact that the thirty-five-year-old woman is likely to be well-groomed, while the younger one may have orange-streaked hair and wear a nose ring. Cosmetic preferences aside, the most noticeable difference between the two women is likely to be the tone of their skin. Despite all the attention lavished on lines, wrinkles, and furrows, skin tone remains one of the most notable differences among youth, middle age, and old age for all skin types and colors.

Healthy skin tone projects youthfulness, vitality, energy, and soundness of mind and body. It is hard to come by through external treatments, although these do have their value. Great skin tone is predominantly a function of the health of the skin—a smooth and translucent epidermis and a strong, undamaged, supportive dermis. The skin's health in turn is intertwined with the health of the body; as the largest organ of the body, the skin is a mirror of your overall health.

All the characteristics of beautiful skin — smoothness, firmness, plumpness, elasticity, and healthy skin tone — ensue from properly nourished skin. The skin cells need nutrients supplied via the blood to function. The more nutrients you keep sending to those cells, the healthier your skin is going to be, and the fresher and more radiant your complexion will be. Even minor nutritional deficiencies can affect the health and appearance of the skin by impairing its ability to renew itself. People who improve their dietary habits often find that their skin tone becomes more youthful, and signs of aging may recede.

In fact, if you want to undertake a journey to the fountain of youth, you need travel no farther than the produce section of your local supermarket. Fruits and vegetables are not only loaded with vitamins and minerals, they are also a rich source of biologically active plant chemicals, known as phytochemicals, that play key roles in cellular activity, repair, and renewal. Scientists have already identified thousands of phytochemicals, and more are being discovered every day. Fruits and vegetables also fortify the body's own natural armor against free radicals — possibly making them one of the very best defenses against disease and aging.

THE MECHANISMS OF AGING

While the exact causes of aging are unknown, researchers now believe that aging starts at the microscopic level of the body, that is, at the level of each individual cell. Damage inflicted at the cellular level causes minute molecular impairments, which over time result in the breakdown of bodily structures and functions associated with aging.

Free radical attacks are one of the most common causes of cellular damage. Lifestyle habits are such a powerful force for

Spotlight on Research

CAN DIET AFFECT SKIN WRINKLING?

Does food and nutrient intake correlate with skin wrinkling? This was the conclusion of one study that looked at the degree of wrinkling of sun-exposed skin in 450 subjects of Greek and Swedish ancestry living in different parts of the world and eating different diets.

Researchers correlated the frequency with which certain foods were eaten with the amount of wrinkling present in an area of the skin that had been exposed to the sun. Subjects with a higher intake of olive oil, fish, vegetables, and legumes and a lower intake of butter, margarine, dairy, and sugar products had less skin damage. A high intake of vegetables, legumes, and olive oil afforded the greatest protective effect. In contrast, subjects who ate a lot of meat, dairy, and butter tended to display greater skin damage.

health or disease because your habits affect the free radical balance of the body—for better or worse. Healthy habits prevent formation of free radicals and bolster the body's natural defenses against free radical attacks. Conversely, unhealthy habits, such as smoking, excess alcohol assumption, eating junk food, poor nutrition, and excessive stress, all increase the oxidative load on the body. The greater the number of free radicals unleashed in the body, the more damage caused.

The skin is particularly susceptible to free radical attacks, because it is rich in lipids, proteins, and DNA, all of which are extremely sensitive to oxidative damage.

The most deleterious effect of free radical attacks, in the skin and elsewhere, is damage to cells' DNA. The cells have their own DNA repair mechanisms, but when free radical assaults get too intense, these mechanisms are unable to keep up. The result is extensive cellular damage. The cumulative effects of this microscopic damage show up as the macroscopic changes we associate with chronic diseases and aging.

Long before free radical damage culminates in a full-fledged health problem, however, the cumulative molecular impairments will affect both your well-being and appearance. Take the example of the circulatory system, one of the body's most vital infrastructures. The blood vessels and millions of fine capillaries of the circulatory system transport nutrient- and oxygen-rich blood to every cell of the body and carry away waste products. Free radical damage, however, contributes to atherosclerosis, which in turn restricts circulation. While the end result of this process can be a heart attack or stroke, there are immediate consequences as well. An impaired circulatory system puts stress on the whole body, impeding its ability to transport vital nutrients needed for its functioning. Insufficient nutrient supply also affects the skin's appearance; the complexion loses color and gradually takes on the grayish tint of oxygen- and nutrient-starved cells.

The body has its own molecular army to defend against free radical attacks. These are *antioxidants*, which neutralize free radicals by giving up electrons without suffering damage themselves. There are two groups of natural antioxidants. The first consists of a number of enzymes largely manufactured by the body itself, such as superoxide dismutase (SOD), catalase, and glutathione peroxidase. The second group consists of antioxidants supplied from food. These include antioxidant vitamins, such as vitamins A, C, and E, coenzyme Q10, selenium, and numerous phytochemicals.

The following chart lists some key nutritional players that can help ward off free radical damage, slow the progression of aging, and enhance your overall appearance.

Anti-Aging, Skin-Friendly Nutrients

VITAMIN A

There are two forms of vitamin A; retinoids and carotenoids. Retinoids are active forms of vitamin A supplied "ready-made" in food. Carotenoids are precursors of vitamin A, which means that the body converts them into vitamin A during the metabolic process. The carotenoid family has more than 600 members, of which beta-carotene is the most well-known.

Benefits for the Skin. The vitamin A family reduces free radical damage induced by UV radiation and protects the skin from age-associated damage. It also brings about the differentiation of skin cells, aids skin repair, and is a key nutrient for numerous skin functions.

Other Health Benefits. Key antioxidant vitamins, vitamin A, and the carotenoids protect against free radical-induced aging. They also prevent cancer and promote healthy eyesight.

Daily Value. 5,000 international units (IU) or 3 mg beta-carotene; too great an intake of vitamin A can result in toxicity and liver damage.

Best Food Sources.
Vitamin A: Dairy products, eggs, salmon, halibut
Carotenoids: Green, leafy vegetables, particularly spinach, kale, broccoli, asparagus, and chard; also yams, carrots, pumpkins, tomatoes, turnips, apricots, peaches, papaya, prunes, cherries, and cantaloupe

B-COMPLEX

Benefits for the Skin. The vitamins of this family are key for skin health. They enhance the complexion and facilitate production of energy in the skin's cells. Vitamin B_2 helps in the production and repair of body tissues, including the skin. Deficiency in this vitamin is often associated with skin damage, including dermatitis. Vitamin B_3 is essential for maintaining healthy skin; it improves blood circulation and skin tone. Vitamin B_{12} provides important nourishment for rapidly dividing cells, including skin cells, and vitamin B_9, or folic acid, is important for cell division and maturation; it also helps the body form red blood cells.

Other Health Benefits. The B-vitamins catalyze the energy production of cells and facilitate production of enzymes needed for extracting energy from food. B_1 helps convert glucose into energy. Deficiency of this vitamin is associated with loss of alertness, heart damage, and respiratory problems.

(Continued on next page)

Anti-Aging, Skin-Friendly Nutrients
(continued)

B_6 curbs inflammation, facilitates formation of red and white blood cells, helps to produce insulin, and enhances immunity. It also plays an important role in emotional balance and memory functions. B_{12} is essential for proper nervous system functioning, including brain and nerve cells. Deficiency might be associated with decay of cognitive capacities.

Suggested Daily Intake.

B_1: 1.1–1.2 mg B_2: 1.1–1.3 mg B_3: 14–16 mg B_6: 2 mg B_9 (folic acid): 180–200 mcg (400 mcg. for childbearing women) B_{12}: 2 mcg

After the age of forty, the body gradually loses its ability to absorb several types of vitamin B, particularly B_6 (from age forty up) and B_{12} (from age sixty up).

Best Food Sources.

Vegetables: Baked potatoes (with their skin), broccoli, collard greens, spinach, avocado, mushrooms, carrots, sweet potatoes, cabbage, brussels sprouts
Fruits: Bananas, apples, figs, citrus fruits
Grains: Oatmeal, rice bran, wheat germ, whole grains
Nuts: Almonds, sunflower and sesame seeds, peanuts, walnuts
Legumes: Beans, lentils
Animal sources: Eggs, chicken, salmon, tuna, mackerel
Other: Brewer's yeast, algae

VITAMIN C

Benefits for the Skin. Plays a key role in the renewal and repair of bodily tissues, including the skin; essential for the formation of collagen.

Other Health Benefits. A key antioxidant vitamin, vitamin C prevents free radical-induced chronic diseases. It also helps to lower levels of "bad" low-density lipids (LDL) cholesterol and increase levels of the "good" HDL cholesterol. It slows atherosclerosis, helps to lower blood pressure, supports immune system functioning, and prevents age-related eye diseases, such as cataracts, glaucoma, night blindness, and age-related macular degeneration.

Suggested Daily Intake. The recommended daily allowance (RDA) of vitamin C is 60 mg, but some nutritionists recommend much higher doses, as much as 1,000 mg a day, to achieve the full anti-aging effects of vitamin C.

Best Food Sources.

Vegetables: Leafy green vegetables, broccoli, asparagus, parsley, cabbage, tomato, potato, peppers, brussels sprouts
Fruits: All fruits, especially citrus fruits, berries, cranberries, kiwi, papaya, melon

(Continued on next page)

Anti-Aging, Skin-Friendly Nutrients
(continued)

VITAMIN E

There are two families of vitamin E: the tocopherol family and the tocotrienols. Tocotrienols were discovered only recently and promise to have the most health-protective and anti-aging benefits of the two families.

Benefits for the Skin. Vitamin E helps to hydrate the skin, reduces inflammation, and aids in healing damaged tissue.

Other Health Benefits. Vitamin E is an important antioxidant vitamin, and it also helps to lower cholesterol level, improves blood flow and circulation, prevents stroke-causing blood clots, and protects against cancer and heart disease.

Suggested Daily Intake. RDA is 40 IU. To reap the full anti-aging benefits of vitamin E, some researchers recommend a daily intake of at least 400 IU. To get this much vitamin E, you have to take supplements; it is not possible to get it from your diet.

Best Food Sources.
Grains: Wheat germ, whole grains
Vegetables: Leafy green vegetables, broccoli, avocado, sweet potatoes
Fruits: Mango
Nuts: Almonds, sunflower seeds, pine nuts
Legumes: Soy beans and soy products
Oils: Most vegetable oils, especially corn oil, sunflower oil
Animal products: Salmon, fish oil

COPPER, SELENIUM, ZINC

Benefits for the Skin. These three minerals work with the antioxidant vitamins to protect cells against free radical damage. In addition, copper is involved in the synthesis of collagen; and zinc facilitates the replacement of old, damaged collagen, promotes cell reproduction, and helps to repair wounds and heal acne.

Other Health Benefits. These three minerals optimize antioxidant vitamin protection to slow aging and protect against chronic diseases. They also facilitate production of antioxidant enzymes and are co-factors in the production of many important enzymes and hormones.

Suggested Daily Intake. Selenium: 70 mcg, copper: 2 mg, zinc: 15 mg; all three trace minerals can be toxic in high doses.

Best Food Sources.
Grains: Wheat germ, whole grains, bran
Dairy: Yogurt, milk

(Continued on next page)

Anti-Aging, Skin-Friendly Nutrients (continued)

Vegetables: Mushrooms, artichokes, broccoli
Nuts: Brazil nuts, walnuts, other nuts and seeds
Legumes: Beans, tofu
Animal products: Chicken, fish, eggs
Other: Blackstrap molasses

COENZYME Q10

Coenzyme Q10 is an important antioxidant and a "biomarker" for aging. Low levels of CoQ10 are correlated with aging and degenerative diseases. CoQ10 is produced by the body itself, but its production declines with age, predisposing the body to chronic oxidative stress and accelerated aging. Nutritionists recommend supplementing with 30–90 mg a day after age fifty.

Benefits for the Skin. Protects against UV-induced free radical damage.

Other Benefits. Defends against free radical damage to the cells' outer protective membrane; assists in cellular metabolism and increases the cells' energy production and capacity to heal; and protects heart health and prevents the proliferation of cancer cells.

Suggested Daily Intake. 30–60 mg/day

Best Food Sources. *Nuts:* Peanuts
Oils: Wheat germ oil, soy oil
Animal products: Salmon, eggs, lean beef, liver, heart, kidneys

ALPHA LIPOIC ACID

A substance manufactured by the body itself, this important antioxidant is also available through supplements.

Benefits for the Skin. Alpha lipoic acid prevents inflammation-induced free radical damage in the skin. It also stimulates enzymatic collagen repair, curbs glycation, and protects against cross-linking, thereby reducing collagen damage.

Other Benefits. Both water- and fat-soluble, this versatile antioxidant can fight free radicals in any part of the cell, making it a potent free radical scavenger. It recycles and renews vitamins C and E, restoring their antioxidant power; assists in cellular metabolism and increases cells' energy production and capacity to heal; regulates blood sugar levels; and may be involved in nerve regeneration.

Suggested Daily Intake. 50–100 mg a day. People with diabetes or nerve damage should talk to their doctor before taking alpha lipoic acid supplements.

Your daily intake of food is one of the most important avenues for fortifying your antioxidant defenses. The greater the number of antioxidants you have floating around in your body at any given time, the greater protection you enjoy against age-accelerating free radical damage. This is why food is such a potent tonic for health and beauty.

New Kids on the Block

Ounce for ounce, fruits and vegetables pack far more antioxidant power than any other type of food. Eating a healthy diet does more than preserve or restore a youthful appearance. A diet rich in fruits and vegetables is well documented as one of the best defenses against age-related chronic diseases, including heart disease, cancer, and stroke. To tap into the anti-aging potential of fruits and vegetables, you need to eat at least five, and ideally ten, servings a day.

Fruits and vegetables are also a rich source of phytochemicals, biologically active plant chemicals that play key roles in bodily repair and renewal. Phytochemicals are a recent arrival on the nutritional scene; they represent one of the most exciting findings in nutrition within the last two decades. Phytochemicals (*phyto* means plant) are not considered essential nutrients; that is, the body does not depend on them for its survival. However, from a preventive standpoint, they are just as vital as vitamins, minerals, and other essential nutrients. Think of them as nutritional medicine. In addition to their powerful antioxidant action, phytochemicals possess numerous healing benefits. You won't develop symptoms of deficiency if you don't get enough phytochemicals, but you will be more vulnerable to aging before your time and developing a chronic or life-threatening disease.

The color, flavor, and scent of vegetables and fruits result from their unique combination of phytochemicals. The easiest way to ensure that you get the full complement of these important substances in your food is to eat a variety of colorful vegetables and fruits every day. Choose foods with the deepest color possible. The deeper the color, the greater the amount of nutrients in the food — be they vitamins, minerals, or phytochemicals. To get a full complement of nutrients from your food, include fruits and vegetables from all color groups — green, red, orange/yellow, and blue/purple.

The Food Pyramid: Roadmap for a Skin-Healthy Diet

Eating five to ten servings of fruits and vegetables daily is the easiest way to start reaping the anti-aging benefits of foods, but there is a lot more to skin-friendly eating. The food pyramid created by the U.S. Department of Agriculture (USDA) provides a good rule of thumb for ensuring that you get the proper nutrients in the right amounts. Here is a guided tour through the latest information available about how different components of the diet affect the skin.

Carbohydrates. Carbohydrates, in the form of glucose (sugar), serve much the same role as gasoline in a car — they supply the fuel needed to run the machinery of the body. Carbohydrates are a vital component of a healthy diet and should constitute some 50 to 60 percent of your daily calorie intake.

Not all carbohydrates are created equal, however. Scientists have created the glycemic index to measure how quickly the glucose of specific foods is broken down and released into the bloodstream. Foods ranking high on the glycemic index cause blood sugar levels to rise quickly, while foods low on the glycemic index do not cause such dramatic swings in blood sugar levels.

Ask the Doctor:

THE ROLE OF SUPPLEMENTS

Q. I find the research on supplements very confusing. First we're told that supplementing with certain nutrients, such as beta-carotene, proects against cancer and other diseases. Then we're told they don't. What's the real story?

A. Taking supplements may seem like an ideal way to reap the anti-aging and cancer-protective benefits of vitamins, minerals, and other vital nutrients. Unfortunately, it's not that simple. It is hard to reproduce the full effects of a given nutrient through supplements. Many vitamins aren't one single substance, but rather families of related substances. There are at least seven different forms of vitamin C and four forms of vitamin E, for example. The carotenoid family, the cancer-protective vitamin A precursors, is made up of at least six hundred members. In short, taking a supplement that provides only one form of a nutrient may not produce the expected result.

Furthermore, nutrients work synergistically; it is most often the *combination* of nutritional substances that confers health benefits. A supplement that isolates specific compounds is less likely to provide such synergistic effects. Supplements might even produce unexpected results. Beta-carotene, for example, increases the body's vitamin E needs, so if you take beta-carotene supplements without also taking an appropriate amount of additional vitamin E, you cannot rule out a negative net health effect.

This is not to say that supplements should be avoided. In combination with a good diet, they definitely serve a purpose. The body's metabolism decreases over time, reducing caloric needs and making it more difficult to get all the nutrients we need through our food. In addition, with advancing age, the body loses part of its ability to absorb or synthesize vital nutrients, such as vitamin E and coenzyme Q10, while the need for antioxidant protection increases.

Taking a multivitamin and mineral supplement can help ensure that you meet your body's basic nutritional needs. A good multi should contain 100 percent of the RDA of as many essential vitamins and minerals as possible (no one multi includes them all). It also makes a lot of sense to take supplements that provide the nutrients not typically found in a multi, such as coenzyme Q10 and essential fatty acids. But remember, supplements should never become an excuse for skimping on the quality of your diet. They can never provide the benefits you get by eating a healthy

How Does Your Diet Measure Up?

To get a general idea of whether your daily diet supplies you with the nutrients you need, check to see if you get enough daily servings of various food groups. For each food group, check off the number in the column that best characterizes your average daily intake of each type of food:

On average, every day I get the following number of servings of:

	I	II	III
Whole grain breads, cereals or other whole grain	❏ 0–3	❏ 4–7	❏ 8+
Vegetables	❏ 0	❏ 1–3	❏ 4–5+
Fruits	❏ 0	❏ 1–2	❏ 3–4+
Meat	❏ 3+	❏ 2	❏ 0–1
Meat alternatives (fish, poultry, nuts, beans)	❏ 0	❏ 1	❏ 2+
Milk or milk products	❏ 0	❏ 1	❏ 2+

For each check in column I, give yourself 0 points; for each check in column II, give yourself 3 points; and for each check in column III, give yourself 5 points.

Score:

0–10 points. Your diet needs improving! Eating a healthier diet will do wonders for your appearance and make you feel better physically, mentally, and emotionally.

10–17 points. Your diet doesn't quite measure up. You and your skin would benefit from eating more (or less) of the food groups in which you got a low score.

18–24 points. You are doing well, but don't rest on your laurels. There is still room for improvement if you are to reap the full benefits of a healthy diet.

25–30 points. Congratulations! You're doing well; keep it up!

To get a more accurate picture of how your diet measures up, go to the USDA's interactive website at www.usda.gov/cnpp/. Answer the questions about your diet, and the site will give you a complete nutritional analysis, free of charge.

High blood sugar levels are dangerous to your health. A diet rich in high-glycemic foods has been linked to diabetes, obesity, impaired immunity, breast cancer, and cardiovascular disease. High blood sugar levels also wreak havoc on the skin's cells and tissues. Collagen and elastin, the two major structural proteins, are particularly vulnerable. When glucose reacts with these proteins (a process called glycation), it causes cross-linking of collagen. There are two types of cross-linking, one healthy and one abnormal. The first is a natural part of collagen formation, and it contributes to the structural strength of collagen. The abnormal cross-linking induced by glycation, however, is accidental and unregulated, and it causes the tissues to harden and lose their flexibility. Abnormal collagen cross-linking is a major factor in the appearance of wrinkles and other types of disruption of skin functions and structure.

Because collagen is present in all types of tissues, glycation-induced cross-linking produces numerous other problems, such as painful joints, accelerated atherosclerosis, and diminished eyesight. Cross-linking in the brain is thought to hamper communication between brain cells, slowing down thought processes and causing memory and concentration problems.

As we grow older, the effect of foods on blood sugar levels becomes even more important, because the body loses some of its ability to regulate these levels. An estimated 50 percent of the population suffers from mildly high blood sugar, also known as glucose intolerance or carbohydrate intolerance.

The most popular foods in our culture — white bread, sugary cereals, pizza, cookies, cakes, sodas, and other processed foods — all contain high-glycemic carbohydrates, which flood the body with glucose molecules minutes after they are eaten. (The average twelve-ounce can of soda alone contains eight teaspoons of sugar.) All these foods have also been linked to decreased insulin sensitivity, which means they impair the body's most important glucose-regulating mechanism. To save your skin — and your long-term health — favor foods that are low on the glycemic index.

TABLE 5.1

The Glycemic Index

FOODS LOW ON THE GLYCEMIC INDEX	FOODS HIGH ON THE GLYCEMIC INDEX
GRAINS, LEGUMES	
Oatmeal (steel-cut)	White flour, white bread
Whole-grain pasta	White pasta
Whole wheat couscous	Pancakes, cookies, other items made with white flour
Soybeans	Corn, corn chips, cornflakes
Chickpeas	Processed cereals with sugar
Lima beans, navy beans	Rice
Rye (whole-grain)	
Lentils	
VEGETABLES	
Yams	Potatoes
Green beans	Carrots
Asparagus	Parsnips
Cabbage	
Leafy greens, such as spinach, kale, chard	
Avocado	
Bell peppers	
Tomatoes	
Broccoli	
FRUITS	
Apples	Fruit juices
Pears	Ripe bananas
Plums	Ripe mangoes
Peaches	Ripe papaya
Cherries	
Citrus fruits	
Melon	
Kiwi fruit	
Blueberries	

Some healthy foods, such as carrots, bananas, and potatoes, rank high on the glycemic index. Instead of avoiding these foods altogether, eat them with low-glycemic foods to balance the overall effect of the meal.

Increase your intake of whole grains to at least three servings a day. Whole grains not only rank favorably on the glycemic index, they may actually improve glucose metabolism and prevent impaired glucose tolerance from progressing to insulin resistance and diabetes. Good sources of whole grain include whole wheat, whole barley, whole oats, cracked wheat, quinoa, bulgar, and whole cornmeal.

Dietary Fiber. Dietary fiber works hand in hand with low-glycemic foods to regulate glucose metabolism. High-fiber foods take longer to break down, and as a result, the glucose they contain is released more gradually into the bloodstream. Dietary fiber is also essential for digestive health. Although it doesn't supply any nutrients, fiber keeps your digestive tract healthy by pushing toxins and other waste products through the intestines more quickly. Nutritionists believe that low levels of fiber intake also are associated with higher risk of cancer, obesity, and atherosclerosis.

The recommended daily dietary fiber intake is twenty to thirty-five grams, but the average American diet supplies only about fifteen grams a day. If you eat two to three servings of whole

The Informed Consumer

LOOK FOR THE WHOLE GRAIN HEALTH CLAIM
Not all so-called whole grain breads contain enough whole grain to produce beneficial effects. To make sure the ones you buy do, check the package label for the following whole grain health claim: "Diets rich in whole grain foods, and other plant foods and low in total fat, saturated fat, and cholesterol, may help reduce the risk of heart disease and certain cancers."

grain foods a day, along with more than five servings of fruits and vegetables, you will have no problem meeting your daily dietary fiber needs.

Skin-Healthy Fats. If you find fats to be a perplexing subject, you are not alone. While some fats are bad for us, others are vital for nourishing the body and the skin, and it can be hard to remember which is which.

A simple rule of thumb for choosing skin-healthy fats is to minimize your intake of saturated fat and favor both types of unsaturated fat, *monounsaturated* and *polyunsaturated*. Saturated fat is found mostly in animal products, such as meat, poultry, milk, and butter; it is also present in such vegetable oils as coconut, palm, and palm kernel oil. This type of fat increases blood levels of LDL cholesterol (the bad type) and total cholesterol, which has been linked to clogging of the arteries and heart disease. Clogging of the arteries also results in diminished blood flow to the skin, producing unhealthy color, fragile skin, and other skin-related problems.

Saturated fat is also thought to promote inflammation, which accelerates the body's aging by increasing the level of free radicals in the body. It also appears to be involved in the so-called fatty degenerative diseases, in which fat appears in parts of the body where it does not belong. This type of dysfunction is implicated in a wide range of health problems, including acne, eczema, allergies, arthritis, gallstones, obesity, and immune system dysfunction. In short, it's smart anti-aging eating to reduce your intake of saturated fat. Nutritionists recommend that you get no more than 30 percent of your daily calories from fat, and fewer than one-third of these should be from saturated fats.

The largest share of your fat consumption should consist of monounsaturated fats, the healthiest type of fat. A diet high in monounsaturated fat reduces the risk of heart disease and breast cancer, it improves cognitive function and prevents memory loss, and it is thought to promote endurance and weight regulation.

The Informed Consumer

BEWARE OF TRANS-FATS

Trans-fats are a special class of "manufactured" fats, which are unlike any of the natural fats found in foods. Listed on product labels as "partially hydrogenated" oils, trans-fats are used in ready-made foods, such as baked goods, chips, crackers, fried foods, frozen dinners, margarine, and shortening.

Trans-fats are even more harmful than saturated fats. They not only increase levels of LDL cholesterol, they also decrease levels of "good" HDL cholesterol. Trans-fats are thought to predispose a person to heart disease, impaired immune function, and cancer. They may also promote inflammation, increase free radical generation, and speed aging processes in the body and the skin.

By some estimates, Americans on average consume one hundred pounds of trans-fats a year, which is no surprise, since most processed foods contain partially hydrogenated oils. To find ready-made foods without trans-fats, check out the health food section of your local supermarket.

In addition, polyunsaturated fats contain omega-3 essential fatty acids (EFAs), a type of fatty acids that is vital for body and skin health. A lack of EFAs may manifest as dry skin, cracked nails, and lifeless hair. It may also cause symptoms of ill health, ranging from digestive disturbances to a lack of energy, depression, and memory problems.

It can be hard to get enough EFAs from your diet, and many nutritionists recommend taking supplements containing flax, borage, evening primrose, or fish oil, all of which are rich sources of EFAs.

Best Bets for Healthy Fats

Monounsaturated Fats. Found in vegetables, such as olive, almond, avocado, peanut, and canola oils. Also present in avocados and nuts, such as pecans, almonds, cashews, walnuts, and peanuts. Monounsaturated oils can be heated to a wide range of cooking temperatures without going bad.

Polyunsaturated Fats. Found in seafood and light vegetable oils such as safflower, soybean, sunflower, corn, sesame, and flaxseed oils. Oils containing polyunsaturated fats go rancid very easily, so use only polyunsaturated oils that have not been exposed to excessive heat, light, or air. Whenever possible, buy expeller-pressed, unrefined oils, because other extraction processes may generate heat and adversely affect the oil. Avoid overheating this type of oil; if it starts smoking, it's too hot.

Omega-3 fatty acids are also found in walnuts, flaxseed, sardines, herring, mackerel, bluefish, tuna, salmon, pilchard, and butterfish. (Avoid cooking fish on high heat, which will destroy much of the omega-3 fatty acids.)

Proteins. Proteins are involved in a vast array of growth, maintenance, and repair functions. There are countless types of proteins, some of which function as hormones, some as enzymes, and some as antibodies, while others facilitate transportation of oxygen and nutrients to all parts of the body. Collagen is one of the essential proteins of the body.

The body creates many of the proteins it needs from amino acids, which are linked together in specific sequences to form different types of proteins. There are twenty amino acids; the body can make twelve of them on its own, but the remaining eight must be supplied from your diet.

There is evidence that a diet that emphasizes plant protein above animal protein affords the greatest anti-aging benefits. Meat is rich in complete protein, but it is also high in saturated fat and cholesterol. The least harmful sources of animal protein are poultry, fish, and lean beef. Plant proteins are easier to digest and may even lower cholesterol. The best sources of plant protein include whole grains and beans. Unlike meat, plants do not provide the full range of amino acids, so you need to eat a variety of plant foods to be sure you get a complete supply of amino acids. The one exception is soy protein, which provides complete protein. Soy foods also contain numerous other health benefits (for more on this, see chapter 6).

Last But Not Least: Don't Forget about Water

While not technically a nutrient, water is essential for bodily functioning, and it happens to be a natural preventive against wrinkles. When the skin loses moisture content, fine lines and wrinkles become more pronounced; if a lot of moisture is lost, the skin becomes dry and flaky. Water helps to hydrate the skin from the inside out.

Water also confers numerous health benefits. It ranks with fiber as an essential component of digestive health—it is needed to make waste move through the system more quickly and effectively. Drinking too little water can predispose you to constipation, headaches, obesity, kidney stones, and even cancer.

It is easy to be mildly dehydrated without knowing it. Unlike hunger, the body's thirst signals are not that effective—you may be short as much as 5 percent of the body's water needs before you start feeling thirsty. Even a little water shortage can cause health problems, since water is essential for numerous bodily processes.

Many nutritionists recommend drinking eight to ten eight-ounce glasses of water a day. Soda, milk, juice, or caffeinated beverages don't count. In fact, both coffee and tea have a diuretic action, causing you to lose more water. If you drink coffee, tea, or other caffeinated beverages, increase your daily water intake by the same amount to make up for the increased water loss.

Well-balanced lifestyle habits are among the best investments you can make in your long-term health and beauty. No amount of money spent on skin care products, rejuvenating therapies, cosmetic surgery, or other anti-aging skin treatments will do as much for the appearance of your skin over the long term as the simple act of maintaining healthy daily habits. You may not be able to turn the clock back twenty years, as wildly enthusiastic anti-aging professionals claim. However, by eating a healthy diet, getting enough exercise and rest, and avoiding excessive stress, you can slow the rate of wear and tear on your body and shave years off your appearance. Even better—you will feel younger too!

CHAPTER 6

Curbing Hormonal Aging

*S*usan arrived for her first consultation with an unusual request: she did not want to end up looking like her hairdresser. "I don't know what's happening to the woman," Susan exclaimed. "She's getting wrinkles so fast, it's like watching a plum left to dry in the sun. She looks a year older each time I see her, and I go there every two months!"

It took a bit of questioning to understand what Susan was talking about, but it soon became clear that her hairdresser was going through menopause. As happens to many women in the years before and after menopause, the hairdresser's skin was losing firmness and elasticity with frightening speed. Every time Susan went to see her, she had more wrinkles around her eyes, more sagging of her jowls, deeper lines around her mouth. In the course of a year, Susan explained, the woman's face had become almost transformed.

Although Susan was clearly prone to exaggeration, her basic observation of the hairdresser's plight was probably correct. The changes a woman's skin undergoes in the years after the onset of menopause can be nothing short of astounding. While the primary determinants of skin aging are the intrinsic and extrinsic aging factors we've explored in previous chapters, hormonal aging is such a considerable force that some researchers consider it a third skin aging factor.

Skin type plays a major role in the degree to which the skin deteriorates during menopause. Women with skin types I and II, who are already more prone to wrinkles, typically experience the most dramatic changes. Women with the darker and thicker skin of types III, IV, or V tend to undergo less striking changes, but they are still affected. Photoaging also comes into play. In the years around menopause, the cumulative effects of photodamage combine with the estrogen-induced decay of skin structures to cause a massive decline of skin structures during the menopausal years.

Most women enter menopause around age fifty, when the ovaries stop releasing eggs and monthly menstruation ceases. Many women experience menopause-related symptoms as early as five to eight years before the actual cessation of their monthly periods (perimenopause).

The transition is accompanied by a pervasive change in hormone levels, particularly estrogen, as the ovaries' output of estrogen, progesterone, and androgens dramatically decreases. In some women, the fluctuating hormone levels produce unpleasant symptoms in the years before and after menopause, such as hot flashes, night sweats, mood swings, sleep problems, irritability, depression, vaginal dryness, loss of libido, and heavier periods.

The drop in estrogen levels also accelerates skin aging. Estrogen is involved in numerous skin functions, and the cells of the epidermis and dermis, along with the blood vessels that pervade the dermis, are packed with estrogen receptors. All the key markers of skin aging—skin thickness and the structural integrity of collagen fibers and blood vessels are under the influence of estrogen.

One of the most pronounced changes the skin undergoes during menopause is a decline in collagen content. While the thickness of male skin diminishes gradually throughout life, women experience a dramatic thinning of the skin in the years around menopause. According to some estimates, a woman may lose as much as 30 percent of skin collagen in the five years after the onset of menopause. Another common symptom is skin dryness. As estrogen levels drop, the sebaceous glands secrete less sebum, reducing the protective surface film of lipids on the surface of the skin. In addition, the dermal ground substance loses hydration and plumpness as the level of water-binding agents, particularly hyaluronic acid, decreases. The blood flow to the dermis is impaired, leading to a less ample supply of important nutrients.

The visible results of all of these changes are rapidly emerging wrinkles and deeper facial creases. The skin loses its elasticity and becomes looser—you can pull it out further, and it won't snap neatly back into place as quickly as young skin.

All of this adds up. There are few times in a woman's life when her appearance undergoes such a drastic transformation as at the onset of menopause. The good news is that these changes are not entirely beyond your control.

Hormone Replacement Therapy and Skin Aging

Women who experience severe symptoms of discomfort during menopause are sometimes advised to go on a short-term hormone replacement therapy (HRT) regimen. As the name implies, HRT eases severe menopausal discomfort, such as hot flashes, night sweats, and mood swings, by replenishing the body's estrogen levels.

A Hormonal Quartet

Estrogen is just one of a set of important hormones—known as sex hormones—that are released by the ovaries. In our early years, these hormones are responsible for development of the secondary sexual characteristics that distinguish men and women. The main female sex hormones are estrogen and its sidekick, progesterone; the male sex hormones are the androgens, particularly testosterone and androstenedione. Both men and women require complementary levels of hormones from the other sex: men secrete a bit of estrogen, and women secrete small amounts of androgens. The delicate balancing act of finding an optimal HRT regimen involves finding a formula that restores the levels of sex hormones while maintaining their finely tuned balance.

Since estrogen is so important for skin health, one might wonder whether HRT would decrease the rate at which the skin decays during menopause. Indeed, there is considerable evidence that it does. Research suggests that the skin of women on HRT retains its youthfulness to a much greater degree than that of women not on HRT. In one study, for example, women treated with hormone therapy for two to ten years had a 48 percent higher skin collagen content than untreated women of the same age. Other studies have shown that the skin of women on HRT stays structurally stronger and retains more of its resilience and elasticity, preventing the slackness otherwise typical in menopausal skin. HRT may also increase peripheral blood flow, further strengthening the skin's health. Estrogen also preserves the content of water-binding agents, such as hyaluronic acid, in the dermal ground substance, keeping the skin well-hydrated and plump.

The most dramatic results of HRT are seen in menopausal women who have already suffered a substantial loss of skin collagen. In such women, estrogen replacement will actually restore collagen content and erase many of the effects of hormonal aging. For women who have lost little or no collagen, estrogen therapy can prevent future skin decay, but, unfortunately, it won't restore collagen to more youthful levels. Some researchers contend that the positive effects on the skin won't manifest unless the treatment is perfectly calibrated to a woman's needs. Indeed, some studies have indicated that too high or too low levels of estrogen replacement might cause lower levels of collagen.

The Pros and Cons of Hormone Replacement Therapy

With the dramatic increase in life expectancy, today's average women can expect to spend one-third of their lives in menopause. That is a long time, and it gives new importance to the quality-of-life concerns and health risks that many women face in the years following menopause. As the old cliché goes, it's not just important to add years to one's life, but to add life to one's years.

It is no small feat to navigate the physiological transformation brought about by menopause without encountering any adverse health consequences. The drop in estrogen can have a pervasive impact not just on your skin, but on your whole body. Researchers suspect that estrogen deficiency is linked to some of the leading health problems that women experience in the last third of their lives.

For several decades, hormone replacement therapy was heralded as *the* breakthough treatment for menopausal women. HRT was thought not only to relieve menopausal complaints, but also to prevent such common aging-related diseases as heart disease, stroke, osteoporosis, and, possibly, Alzheimer's disease. Still, questions remained, foremost among them the unsettling prospect that HRT might actually increase the risk of contracting uterine cancer.

That all came to an abrupt halt in the summer of 2002, when the largest-ever study of the long-term effects of hormone replacement therapy was stopped three years short of its scheduled completion. The reason? Based on data already collected, researchers concluded that the risks of long-term HRT use outweighed the benefits. The study, which was part of a group of studies known as the Women's Health Initiative (WHI), found that while women on HRT did have decreased incidence of hip fractures (an indication of osteoporosis) and colon cancer, they developed more cases of heart disease, breast cancer, stroke, and blood clots. The researchers felt that the risks of long-term HRT use so clearly outweighed the benefits that it was not advisable to continue the study.

The WHI results caused a dramatic reversal in the medical community's attitude toward HRT. Still, doctors agree, the risks emerge largely with long-term HRT use. For this reason, short-term use of HRT is still a viable option for easing the menopausal transition.

While estrogen's benefits for the skin can be impressive, this obviously should not be the only motivation for going on HRT. HRT is a potent drug, and it is not something to take for purely esthetic reasons. While short-term use is considered to be relatively safe, the longer you stay on the treatment, the greater the risk that it might cause other health problems.

Doctors now agree that there is a strong case for looking at alternatives to HRT. There is increasing evidence that simple lifestyle changes can help reduce menopausal discomfort and lower the risk of developing heart disease, osteoporosis, or

Alzheimer's disease. For many women, this is perhaps the most convincing argument against HRT.

Boosting Hormonal Health

When it comes to alternative ways of navigating hormonal aging, much the same rules apply as for curbing extrinsic aging. Avoid lifestyle factors that increase the stress load on your body, such as smoking and excessive alcohol and caffeine consumption. Add habits that enhance hormonal health and prevent the health problems most commonly related to estrogen deficiency. The simple act of exercising three to five times a week can help to reduce menopausal discomfort, *and* it will boost heart health and protect your bones. Keeping on top of your diet is important as well. Make sure you get enough of the nutrients that you need more of as you age: calcium; B vitamins; antioxidant vitamins A, C, and E; and the trace minerals, copper, selenium, and zinc. Monitor your risk of osteoporosis every two to three years by having a bone density test. Reduce your intake of animal fats and processed foods and include more fruits, vegetables, and whole grains in your diet.

One of the most exciting new areas of menopausal research concerns whether certain plant foods might offer protection against fluctuating hormone levels. These are foods rich in naturally occurring plant estrogens, or phytoestrogens as they are also called. When ingested, these plant compounds exert estrogenlike biological activity in the body by interacting with the body's estrogen receptors and stabilizing hormonal fluctuations. Some researchers believe that phytoestrogens have both estrogenic and antiestrogenic effects, depending on the internal hormonal environment of the body. According to this theory, in menopausal women with low levels of estrogen, phytoestrogens act like estrogen and help to stabilize menopausal symptoms. In premenopausal women with high levels of estrogens, phytoestrogens instead might interact with the cells' estrogen receptors and moderate estrogen levels. Since high estrogen levels over a lifetime are thought to increase the risk of breast cancer, this might protect against this disease.

The main classes of phytoestrogens are *isoflavones*, particularly found in soybeans, and *lignans*, found in flaxseed. Soy has been found to reduce the number of hot flashes in a group of menopausal women, with a 33 percent average reduction after four weeks and a 45 percent reduction after twelve weeks. Other studies have reported as much as a 40 percent decrease in common menopausal symptoms, such as hot flashes, night sweats, headaches, sleep disturbances, fatigue, depression, and loss of libido in women who supplemented their diet with about forty-five grams of soy flour a day (six tablespoons). Eating either two tablespoons of flaxseed or six tablespoons of soy flour a day actually has been found to increase estrogen levels in the blood after two weeks.

Research suggests that plant estrogens in soy and flaxseed may have favorable effects on the cardiovascular system by balancing cholesterol levels as well. Flaxseed is also a rich source of omega-3 essential fatty acids, the healthy type of oil, which provides many heart-protective benefits, including improved circulation, reduced blood clotting, and fewer inflammatory changes.

One of the most well-researched health benefits of soy consumption concerns cancer protection. Researchers first became aware of the potential impact of soy foods on cancer risk by studying disease patterns in Asian populations. In these countries, soy consumption is high and cancer rates are low — including breast, colon, prostate, and endometrial cancer. (Incidentally, the incidence of atherosclerotic diseases, such as heart disease and stroke, is also much lower.) The cancer-preventative benefits of soy might derive from compounds other than isoflavones, including antioxidants and *protease inhibitors,* which are thought to block activation of cancer genes in the colon, lung, pancreas, and breast. Unfortunately, the evidence concerning the effects of phytoestrogens is inconsistent, and some studies have failed to find an effect of dietary intake of phytoestrogens on menopausal symptoms.

Might plant estrogens confer similar benefits on skin aging as hormone replacement therapy? That is the million-dollar question. Our knowledge of phytoestrogens and their effects on the body is still in its infancy, and it would be premature to speculate on any such effects. However, phytoestrogens are present in foods that generally work wonders for the skin, so either way you win. The most abundant sources of phytoestrogen are soy and flaxseed, but they are also prevalent in legumes, such as chickpeas, lima beans, and whole grains, and in many fruits and vegetables. Many herbs that women in traditional cultures take during menopause, such as dong quai, red clover, and chasteberry, also have been found to have high concentrations of plant estrogenic compounds.

To ease menopausal symptoms, you would need a daily intake of 50–150 mg of isoflavones, or two to three servings of soy. According to the University of California Berkeley *Wellness Letter,* it is not advisable to try to get your soy intake through supplements containing isolated soy components, such as isoflavones, because it is still not entirely clear what causes soy's benefits. It is thought to be the two primary soy isoflavones, genistein and daidzein, but it might be other substances in soy — or the combined effect of several substances. In addition, soy powders or concentrates are not desirable sources of soy, since they contain fairly low levels of isoflavones.

The popularity of soy has increased tremendously over the past few years, and many food products based on soy are now available in supermarkets. Tofu, or bean curd, is an old soy staple that is now available as vegetarian burgers, enchiladas, hot dogs, and even ice cream. Flaxseed is another important source of phytoestrogens. The best way to take them is to grind one or two tablespoons in a coffee grinder each day and sprinkle over your food.

Stemming Collagen Loss

In addition to adopting a general menopausal health regimen, there are numerous specific things you can do for your skin to slow hormonal aging. It is particularly important to take steps to prevent collagen loss and facilitate the synthesis of new collagen. Collagen constitutes some 97.5 percent of the fibrous protein of the dermis, while elastin only makes up the last 2.5 percent. Like all components of the body, collagen is constantly being renewed, but as we grow older, the skin gradually loses its ability to replace old collagen, predisposing us to wrinkles.

With the right knowledge and tools, the skin's collagen metabolism can be enhanced in a number of ways. First of all, focus on prevention. Numerous factors increase the rate at which collagen is damaged and worn out. Enter the usual suspects: lifestyle factors that increase the production of free radicals, including environmental toxins, sun damage, and smoking. In addition to increasing oxidative stress in the body, smoking impedes the skin's ability to produce new collagen. According to some studies, synthesis of the main type of collagen in the skin during wound healing is reduced by 18 percent more in smokers than in nonsmokers.

Second, make sure your diet includes plenty of the nutrients essential for collagen formation, such as vitamin C. Signs of impaired collagen synthesis caused by vitamin C deficiency may include poor wound healing, bleeding gums, and skin hemorrhages. Conversely, supplying extra vitamin C in your diet may enhance collagen synthesis, particularly in the presence of other dietary factors that stimulate collagen production. These include certain amino acids, particularly *proline, lysine,* and *glycine* and the trace mineral copper. In addition to its antioxidant functions, copper facilitates collagen production, and it is thought to play a role in certain enzymatic activities involved in collagen and elastin synthesis. Copper is found in raisins, nuts, sweet potatoes, kidney beans, and seafood such as lobster and oysters.

Even exercise, albeit indirectly, may build skin thickness and counteract the ravages of aging. In one study of 146 women, for example, researchers S. Elizabeth Whitmore, MD, and Michael A. Levine, MD, of the departments of Dermatology and Medicine at the Johns Hopkins University found that women who exercised more tended to have thicker skin. Exercise might contribute to thicker skin by increasing blood flow to the skin, providing more oxygen and vital nutrients, and enhancing secretion of human growth hormone. Growth hormone is one of the signal molecules that regulate the activity of the cells. The level of these signal molecules decreases with age, and the decline in human growth hormone in particular is thought to be linked to many of the problems of aging other than wrinkling, including cardiovascular disease, osteoporosis, decreased sexual function, and so on.

Up to this point, we have looked at simple things you can do to protect your skin from the ravages of environmental aging as well as the many ways in which you can enhance the health of the skin from the inside out. This is only half the story, however. There are also numerous ways to augment the appearance of the skin from the outside in. The years before and after the onset of menopause are particularly important, because this is the time to change your daily skin care routine to take into account the special needs of aging skin. You also will want to take a close look at some of the exciting anti-aging treatments that have emerged within the last decade that can actually stimulate the production of new collagen.

These key topics will be the focus of the rest of book. Chapters 7 and 8 lay out skin care techniques that you can apply at home to enhance the health and youthfulness of your skin, stimulate collagen synthesis, and delay the emergence of wrinkles, no matter what your age. Chapters 9 through 12 explore groundbreaking new treatments for restoring skin health and stimulating collagen growth, which literally have the potential to take years off your appearance.

PART III

Caring for Your Skin:
Breakthrough Skin Care Treatments
For Turning Back the Clock

CHAPTER 7

How to Keep Your Skin Looking Its Best at Any Age

*A*t every moment of your life, your skin is exposed to numerous abuses: sunlight, extremes of weather, dietary insufficiencies or indiscretions, pollutants, and various types of external and internal stress. All of these affect the skin over time, causing the texture, firmness, and skin tone changes that we associate with aging.

As we have seen in earlier chapters, you can do a lot to slow age-related deterioration of the skin by maximizing your intake of the nutrients needed for healthy skin function and minimizing exposure to things that damage the skin. In addition, a good skin care routine is essential to make the most of your skin at any age and to defend it against aging. Proper care of the skin will facilitate its natural self-rejuvenating functions and help to protect it against the damaging effects of the sun, environmental pollution, and extremes of weather. It won't make you look like a thirty-four-year-old if you are sixty-four, but it will go a long way toward keeping your skin healthy and youthful.

Zeroing in on a good skin care routine is not rocket science, but it is one area where most women consistently experience great frustration. For many women, the hunt for the right skin care products is a constant crusade. Women are constantly bombarded with advertising claims, each loftier than the previous one. Amid all the marketing hype, it can be hard to know which products perform the functions they promise, which ingredients really do make a difference, and when you're paying a lot for a product that is no more effective than cheaper ones.

Nonetheless, it is worth expending a little effort to navigate through the marketing maze, because good skin care habits should be a key component of your anti-aging repertoire. In this and the following chapter, we lay out the basic knowledge you need to sift through the hype and evaluate the effectiveness of a product, not only on its own merits, but also in terms of how suitable it is for your skin. We also show you how to distinguish between skin care products with known age-defying properties and those that show promise but are still in an early development phase.

Understanding Your Skin's Changing Needs

The common advice for developing a good skin care routine is to determine what your skin type is and learn about its specific needs. Identifying your skin type is easier said than done, however, because it fluctuates over time. The condition of your skin is strongly affected by external factors, such as the climate you are in, the season of the year, your daily skin care habits, and major life transitions, such as pregnancy or menopause.

In short, don't regard your skin type as static—be ready to change skin care strategies as the characteristics of your skin change. You may even have several skin conditions going on at

TABLE 7.1

Characteristics of the Different Skin Types

NORMAL SKIN	DRY SKIN	OILY SKIN	COMBINATION SKIN
•Refined and smooth texture	•Feels tight, particularly after washing	•Feels greasy	•Shiny, oil patches on nose and forehead
•Clear appearance	•Sometimes flaky or itchy	•Shiny appearance	•Normal to dry skin on cheeks and neck
•Neither dry nor oily	•No greasy areas	•Large, visible pores	•Large pores on T-zone
•Supple, elastic	•Looks dull, lifeless	•Prone to blemishes	

the same time. As you grow older, the thin skin around your eyes might become extremely dry and sensitive, while the skin on your forehead continues to be oily and prone to blemishes. In such situations, simply treat each area with the care appropriate for it.

As the skin matures, two themes often become increasingly apparent: the need to preserve moisture and the need to protect your increasingly sensitive skin. Proper moisture content is essential to maintain the elasticity of the skin, keeping it pliable and smooth. Dry skin will cause your skin to feel tight and rough to the touch, and fine lines and wrinkles are more apparent on poorly hydrated skin. Water-deficient skin also becomes more vulnerable to damage and is ruptured more easily.

The skin has numerous built-in moisturizing mechanisms. It is kept hydrated by a constant supply of water delivered by tiny blood vessels in the dermis to the upper layer of the epidermis, the stratum corneum. In addition, the stratum corneum contains a number of substances, which together are known as the skin's *natural moisturizing factor* (NMF), that help retain water content and keep the skin moist and pliable. Further protection against moisture loss is created by lipids, such as ceramides, free fatty acids, and cholesterol. These surround the tightly packed corneocytes of the stratum corneum and trap water molecules, blocking water evaporation and preventing the natural moisturizing factors from escaping out of the surface layers of skin.

After age forty, numerous factors conspire to dry out the top layers of the skin. The concentration of both NMPs and intercellular lipids decreases sharply, impairing the skin's natural hydrating capacity and increasing the propensity for dryness. In addition, the water-holding proteins known as glycosaminoglycans (GAGs) in the dermis decrease in number, causing the skin to lose an important source of hydration. The dermal collagen network, which also retains water, loses some of its moisturizing ability, making it less pliable and resilient.

Dry, maturing skin is also prone to sensitivity and allergic reactions, although all skin types (and all ages) have the potential to be sensitive if exposed to irritating conditions. Skin sensitivity is most prevalent among fair-skinned individuals of skin type I and less common among blacks or dark-skinned individuals.

Sensitive skin is very reactive and easily affected by external stress, including too much sun, cold, rapid temperature changes, or unsuitable cosmetic products. When visible, skin sensitivity shows up as breakouts or as red or blotchy skin. However, often there are no visible signs of skin irritation; the skin simply feels as if it is slightly burning, stinging, or generally delicate. Sensitive skin is also prone to allergic reactions, which appear as rashes, hives, or intense itching.

Skin sensitivity is not something to be taken lightly. Some experts believe that chronic, subclinical inflammation in irritated skin might actually cause long-term damage and accelerate aging. Chronic inflammation damages the cellular environment and may cause abnormal changes in the lower layer of the skin similar to those induced by UV radiation.

Caring for Maturing Skin

If your skin is becoming dry and more sensitive with age, you need to adjust your daily skin care routine accordingly. It becomes particularly important to minimize any external influences that will upset the balance of the skin. Stay clear of cosmetic products with harsh or potentially sensitizing ingredients.

Cleansing remains one of the key ways to enhance the health and appearance of your skin. It removes dust and makeup, dislodges dead skin cells, and facilitates skin turnover. As your skin matures, your daily cleansing regimen should become more gentle. Choose a cleanser that is mild and nondrying, yet able to dissolve old sebum and dislodge old, dead skin cells. If you wear makeup, the cleanser must be able to remove it without scrubbing or rubbing. Make sure the cleanser washes off easily and doesn't leave a filmy residue. If a cleanser leaves your skin feeling dry, it is stripping away the skin's natural moisture-protective mantle. Similarly, if it creates irritation in the form of redness or a slight tingling, the product isn't for you. Avoid highly fragranced products, because perfume ingredients are the most common skin irritants.

Some cleansers include mildly abrasive ingredients, such as ground shells of apricots or almonds, fine sand, or silica, that aim to scrub off dead skin cells and accelerate the skin's natural exfoliating process. The abrasive particles in such cleansers can be sharp and irregular, and they may scratch delicate skin and cause irritation. Newer versions of this type of cleanser use microbeads made of synthetic material that are more uniform in size and not

---

TABLE 7.2
Cleansing Tips for Different Skin Conditions

DRY AND SENSITIVE SKIN

- Use a gentle and nondrying cleanser. Most liquid, milky cleansers work well, or try beauty bars rich in fatty substances, such as cocoa butter, lanolin, or petrolatum.

- Use a cream cleanser that rinses off easily without leaving a residue that has to be removed with a toner, which might irritate the skin.

- Rinse your face thoroughly in lukewarm water. Never use very cold or hot water as this puts stress on the fine capillaries in the skin.

- Avoid facial steamers, steam baths, and saunas; these can aggravate any existing skin irritation.

- Wet washcloths can be hard on sensitive skin, and they are a breeding ground for bacteria. If you're wearing hard-to-remove makeup, try cleansing twice instead of rubbing makeup off with a washcloth.

OILY SKIN

- Use a nondrying cleanser that will get rid of excess oil without stripping the skin of moisture. Oil-based products make good cleansers, because they dissolve sebum. Avoid rich, fatty, or moisturizing soaps.

- Don't use alcohol-based astringent toners and other drying products—these can backfire and cause the oil glands to step up oil production.

- Wash your face no more than 2 or 3 times a day. Excessive washing may irritate the skin and cause the oil glands to produce more oil.

- If your skin is very oily, try using a clay mask or a mask made with milk of magnesia (plain) 1–3 times a week. Like clay, magnesium is an earth mineral, but it absorbs oil more effectively than clay. It may take several applications for results to become apparent.

COMBINATION SKIN

- When cleaning your face, don't just focus on the T-zone area—make sure you cover the whole face. Then follow with a gentle, nonalcohol-based astringent on the T-zone area.

- For an excessively oily T-zone, try using a mask with milk of magnesia (plain) every other day on that part of your face (see Oily Skin, above).

TABLE 7.3

Cleansers Suited for Mature Skin

CETAPHIL GENTLE DAILY CLEANSER

Formulated for dermatologists. It is nondrying and well suited for all skin types, including sensitive skin. Cetaphil is compatible with the skin's natural pH and does not remove the skin's protective oils. If it's not sufficient to remove your makeup, try Cetaphil Daily Facial Cleanser instead.

BIORÉ FOAMING LIQUID CLEANSER

This cleanser is hypoallergenic and noncomedogenic (i.e., nonpore-clogging). It is sufficiently mild for use on dry or sensitive skin, but it can also be used on oily skin.

AQUAFIL

A mild, moisturizing cleanser.

NEUTROGENA EXTRA GENTLE CLEANSER

Nonsoap formula that adds moisture to the skin. The detergent used is one of those least irritating to the skin. Does not remove makeup very well.

---

so harsh on the skin. If you use a chemically exfoliating product containing alpha hydroxy acids (AHAs) and beta hydroxy acids (BHAs) (see chapter 8), there is no need for an abrasive cleanser.

Some cleansers seek to increase exfoliation by including AHAs and BHAs, which might seem to be an appealing alternative to using a separate exfoliating product. Unfortunately, cleansers do not stay on the skin long enough for the exfoliating agents to have any substantial effects. (Cleansers should never be left on the skin for very long, because many contain detergents that will irritate the skin with extended exposure.)

If your skin develops a sensitizing reaction, it can continue for a while even if you stop using the product that triggered it in the first place. During this time, avoid rubbing or scrubbing the skin

The Informed Consumer

THE GREAT SLS DEBATE

Skin cleansers, hair shampoo, and other types of cosmetic cleansing products often contain detergents that are potential skin irritants. In particular, a great deal of debate surrounds the safety of sodium lauryl sulfate (SLS) and its chemical cousin, sodium laureth sulfate (SLES).

The Cosmetic Ingredient Review (CIR), a panel of experts established by the Cosmetic, Toiletry and Fragrance Association together with the FDA review and assess the safety of cosmetic ingredients, has issued a safety alert on the two ingredients.

According to the CIR, both ingredients cause skin irritation in animals and in some humans. SLS may also build up in hair follicles, potentially damaging the follicle and causing hair loss. Sodium laureth sulfate (and its cousin, ammonium laureth sulfate) is somewhat less irritating, because its molecules are larger and less able to penetrate the skin and hair. The CIR asserts that while both ingredients can be skin irritants, the low concentrations of them used in cosmetic products are safe for brief applications.

If you wish to minimize your exposure to these ingredients, look for products that either don't include them or list them toward the end of the ingredient list (an indication that they are not the primary detergents in the product). If you use a cleanser or shampoo with either of these ingredients, be sure to rinse thoroughly; prolonged exposure from residue left on the skin will increase the risk of irritation. If your skin is extremely sensitive, consider avoiding products containing SLS or SLES.

and steer clear of skin care products that are known to cause mild skin irritation, including skin lighteners, AHAs, Retin-A®, or Renova® (see chapter 8), and fragrance-filled products.

If you use a toner, this might also be a time to reevaluate whether you need this type of product. Many toners contain potentially irritating ingredients. Astringent toners, for example, can contain as much as 20 percent alcohol, making them extremely drying and irritating to the skin. Claims that toners can close or tighten your pores or deep clean the skin are all exaggerated. A toner can remove any remaining makeup or soapy residue after you have cleaned and rinsed off your skin; however, you can accomplish much the same thing by using a good cleanser and rinsing your face thoroughly.

If you enjoy the feeling of a toner and don't have sensitive skin, use a gentle, nondrying toner after cleaning your face. Look for toners that contain water-binding and anti-irritant ingredients, such as allantoin, aloe, bisabolol, burdock root, or licorice root. Avoid products that contain alcohol or witch hazel, which dry the skin. You don't have to spend a fortune on a toner. More expensive toners often contain much the same ingredients as less expensive ones.

Moisturizer Magic and Mania

A good moisturizer is your single most important weapon for counteracting escalating skin dryness. Yet, given the number of products on the market and the considerable number launched in any given year, choosing a moisturizer can turn into an immensely frustrating activity. The task is not made any easier by the lofty promises of "proven repair," "dramatically reduced lines, puffiness, and dark circles," "visibly improved skin texture," and "enhanced firmness" that lure women to the cosmetics counter.

No standard moisturizer, no matter how well-formulated it is, has the capacity to remove wrinkles, alter the structure of the skin, or permanently restore its firmness. Nonetheless, a good moisturizer is an important component of a daily skin care regimen, particularly for dry skin. While moisturizers won't erase or

The Informed Consumer

 WHAT'S IN A NAME?
Numerous products on the market purport to address the needs of people with sensitive skin. Unfortunately, there are no regulatory standards for such products, and manufacturers set their own standards. Hypoallergenic products, for example, are defined as products that are less likely to cause allergic reactions. But while some manufacturers might do thorough clinical testing before launching a hypoallergenic product, others might simply leave out some of the most common skin-irritating ingredients. This is also the case for products claiming to be "dermatologist-tested" or "nonirritating."

Fragrance is the most common trigger of allergic reactions. Even if a product claims to be fragrance-free, small amounts of fragrance may still be included to conceal unpleasant odors from other ingredients.

remove wrinkles, they can help to prevent the "prune effect," in which wrinkles appear deeper than they do when the skin is moist. Similarly, a good moisturizer will make the skin more flexible and smoother, and will increase the skin's glow, because its water content augments light reflection.

ANATOMY OF A MOISTURIZER

If you have ever looked at the long list of ingredients on a moisturizer package and felt utterly confused, you are not alone. Fortunately, you don't need a degree in chemistry to understand how moisturizers work, because they are all structured according to the same simple principles. Moisturizers seek to mimic the skin's own moisturizing mechanisms by using ingredients that either *block* the loss of water from the skin or *attract* additional water from the dermis to the surface layers of the skin.

There are two main categories of ingredients in moisturizers. *Occlusive agents* are substances that create an oily barrier on the surface of the skin, which slows the natural evaporation of water from the stratum corneum. Common occlusive ingredients include petrolatum, paraffin, beeswax, and various vegetable and animal fats, such as lanolins, cocoa butter, and jojoba, olive, and almond oils. Occlusives can be heavy and greasy on the skin and can cause breakouts in acne-prone individuals. To avoid this, some moisturizers rely on silicones, such as dimethicone and cyclomethicone, as occlusive agents. Silicones are clear liquids with an oily feel, but without the undesirable, pore-clogging properties of oil. The art of creating a moisturizer involves finding the blend of occlusives that will do the best job of reducing water loss without feeling heavy and greasy on the skin or causing acne breakouts.

Humectant agents increase water content by attrating, natural moisture from the underlying skin tissue. Some humectants can bind up to a thousand times their weight in water. They are lighter than occlusives and don't feel greasy on the skin. Many humectants used in moisturizers, such as urea, lactates, hyaluronic acids, and pyrrolidone carboxylic acid (PCA), occur naturally in the skin.

Other types of ingredients in moisturizers perform related functions. *Emollients* fill in the tiny crevices between the surface skin cells, lubricating the skin and making it softer and smoother. Emollients vary in their degree of greasiness; some are rather light and spread easily on the skin, while others are heavier and have occlusive properties. The "feel" and function of the moisturizer when applied to the skin is determined in part by the emollients included. Cosmetic chemists include lighter emollients in day creams and body lotions, while heavier emollients are used in night and eye creams. Careful selection of emollients is important, because they often interact with other ingredients in the formulation. The absorption spectrum of a sunscreen, for example, may be changed simply by including certain emollients.

Numerous inactive ingredients perform various housekeeping functions. *Preservatives* prevent the growth of bacteria and protect the product from contamination. *Emulsifiers* allow non-mixable liquids — such as the water and oil in a cream or lotion — to blend and stay in suspension rather than separate as oil and water usually do when you mix them together. *Solvents* dissolve other ingredients, facilitating their absorption, while *fragrances* mask any unpleasant odors or add a pleasing and attractive aroma to the product.

Most moisturizers have a high water content, typically between 65 and 85 percent. Water plays several roles: it acts as a hydrating agent, it facilitates absorption of the other ingredients of the moisturizer, and it dilutes and disperses the active and inactive ingredients of the moisturizer. Moisturizers fall into two main groups: oil-in-water formulations and water-in-oil formulations. Oil-in-water formulations contain tiny droplets of oil held in water, giving the moisturizer a lighter, easily absorbed feel. In water-in-oil preparations, the water is held within the oil, giving the formulation a heavier, oilier feel, which stays longer on the surface of the skin. Day creams are typically oil-in-water formulations, while the heavier night creams tend to be water-in-oil. See table 7.4 for common moisturizer ingredients.

HOW TO CHOOSE A MOISTURIZER

How do you choose a moisturizer that is suitable for your skin? It is easy to spend a lot of money on moisturizers. Most skin care companies do a great job of persuading women to spend a fortune on expensive products using alluring packaging and lofty claims. However, save your money; there's no guarantee

TABLE 7.4

Moisturizers—Some Common Ingredients

WATER (65–85%)	LIPIDS (OCCULUSIVES) (5–35%)	HUMECTANTS, EMOLLIENTS (0.5–15%)	OTHER (1.1–3%)
	Hydrocarbon oils and waxes: Petrolatum mineral oil parafin squalene	*Common humectants:* Glycerin Sodium lactate Pyrolidone carboxylic acid Urea Gelatin Propylene glycol Alpha hydroxy acids Sorbitol Hyaluronic acid Some vitamins and minerals	*Emulsifiers (1–2%):* Triethanolaine quaternium 15 stearic acid triethaolamine glyceryl monostearate polysorbates
	Animal fats: lanolin cholesterol		*Preservatives (0.1–1%):* butyl, propyl, ethyl, and methyl parabens, disodium EDTA quarternium 15 imidazolydyl urea methylisothiazoline alcohols trisodium and tetrasocium edetate (EDTA, tocopherol (vitamin E)
	Vegetable oils: cocoa butter coconut oil almond oil oleic acid (olive oil)		
	Fatty acids: lanolin acid stearic acid	*Common emollients:*	
	Silicone: dimethicone cyclomethicone	*Alcohols:* Octyl dodecanol, oleyl alcohol hexyl decanol	
	Fatty alcohol: lanolin alcohol cetyl alcohol	*Esters:* Oleyl oleate isopropyl myristate myristl myristate cetearyl isonomanoate coco caprylate PEG-7 glycerl cocoate octyl stearate	*Fragrances (<.25%):* Synthetic or derived from essential oils
	Waxes: beeswax stearyl stearate lanolin		

You can find more information about ingredients in cosmetics by consulting the *International Cosmetic Ingredient Dictionary*, available at many public libraries.

that a moisturizer that costs $35 or more per ounce is any more effective than one that costs $2 per ounce. The high-priced version may smell better and have a nicer "feel" on the skin, but when it comes to the bottom line—how well it keeps the skin hydrated—many high-priced moisturizers actually perform worse than lower-priced versions.

This has been the conclusion of several studies on moisturizers by *Consumer Reports* over the years. In one study, *Consumer Reports* tested twenty-eight lotions and creams for the face and body. The moisture level of the skin was measured before each cream was applied, and after one hour, two hours, and four hours. In addition, experienced panelists checked the "feel" of the product—its scent, its consistency, how easily it spread on the skin, and whether it disappeared quickly or left a residue.

The effectiveness of the moisturizers varied widely. All of them enhanced moisture levels, but the best ones boosted moisture levels substantially more, and the effects lasted much longer. The moisturizers ranged in price from $1.40 to $33 per ounce, but the five highest-ranked moisturizers were all under $2.50 per ounce. The best of the expensive products ranked sixth and seventh. Body lotions in general had less effective moisturizing capability than facial moisturizers. In addition, products formulated specifically for African-American skin performed no better for that skin tone than those formulated for all skin tones.

WHEN TO USE A MOISTURIZER

It's commonly believed that you need to use a moisturizer to prevent wrinkles, but that is not at all the case. Moisturizers can temporarily reduce fine lines in dry skin and smooth the skin. However, if you have oily skin, or if you are prone to breakouts, a moisturizer may do more harm than good. Even for normal skin, a moisturizer may not be needed, while people with combination skin should use it only on dry areas.

If moisturizers are overused, or applied to skin that is sufficiently hydrated already, they can disrupt the skin's normal function. Studies have shown, for example, that if the hydration level of the stratum corneum is increased with moisturizers in other-

The Informed Consumer

THE FDA AND THE COSMETICS INDUSTRY
The reason it is so hard to untangle truth from fiction when it comes to cosmetics products is that the cosmetics industry is not subject to the same stringent regulations as the drug industry. While the Food and Drug Administration requires drugs to undergo rigorous testing to assess their effectiveness and safety before they are approved for general use, no such requirements apply to cosmetics and skin care products. The FDA relies on cosmetics manufacturers to do their own quality control and product testing.

This makes for a triple whammy for consumers. First, of the more than five thousand cosmetics ingredients, few have been tested for their long-term safety and effects on the skin. Second, products may be touted as new, breakthrough skin care miracles, but in reality, their effects on the skin are not backed by solid research. Third, even when products do contain ingredients with scientifically verified effects, the ingredients are not necessarily present in a sufficient concentration to produce the promised results, or they may have lost their potency by the time they reach the consumer.

wise normal skin, the efficiency of the skin's own natural barrier is impaired. This in turn increases the skin's susceptibility to irritants, because the stratum corneum becomes more permeable to irritating agents. Also, excessive use of moisturizers, especially ones that are too heavy for your skin, can clog pores, predisposing you to breakouts.

So if your skin isn't dry, you don't necessarily need a moisturizer. The main idea is not to overburden your skin with cosmetic

TABLE 7.5
Moisturizing Tips for Different Skin Conditions

DRY SKIN

- Immediately before applying a moisturizer, spray your face with a fine mist of water or rosewater—or simply apply the moisturizer while your skin is still damp after washing. The moisturizer will seal the water into the skin, further increasing hydration.
- If your skin is very dry, look for moisturizers rich in hydrating ingredients, both occlusives and humectants. Use a day cream with an SPF of 15 and a heavier cream at night.
- Skin loses a lot of water to the air, particularly in the winter, when indoor humidity can drop to as low as 5 or 10 percent. Install a whole-house humidifier, or at the very least, keep a humidifier or a cool-mist vaporizer in your bedroom.
- Never, ever, venture out on a cold or windy winter day without a protective layer of moisturizer on your face. Cold and wind will dry out unprotected skin in no time.

SENSITIVE SKIN

- Pick a moisturizer with fewer than ten ingredients. The fewer the ingredients, the less the potential for irritation.
- Look for moisturizers without standard irritating ingredients, such as fragrance, lanolin, propylene glycol, or formaldehyde-releasing preservatives, such as quaternium 15.
- When trying out new cosmetic products, test them first by applying to a small patch of skin and wait to see if any reaction (redness, itching) develops.

OILY SKIN

- Your skin doesn't necessarily need a moisturizer. If you want to use one, opt for one that is light and lists water as its first ingredient. Alternatively, pick one that is oil-free (using silicones instead of oil). Whenever you go out, use an oil-free sunscreen with an SPF of 15.
- Use an oil-free powder or foundation to reduce oily shine—but don't overdo it! Too much foundation or powder makes skin appear chalky.
- Stay clear of moisturizers that contain rich emollients, such as cocoa butter, oleic acid, linseed, peanut, or sesame oil.

COMBINATION SKIN

- A good moisturizer can help balance combination skin. Use a moisturizer primarily in the dry areas where you really need it, keeping it away from the oily T-zone.
- Use mild products for sensitive areas of dry skin. If you use stronger products on the oily areas, be sure to keep them away from the dry areas of your face.
- If you use makeup, switch to an oil-free foundation if a standard water-based one doesn't work for the oily areas of your face.

products that you don't really need. As the skin matures and becomes more dry, the need for moisturizers generally increases. You may also need a heavier and oilier type of moisturizer and more frequent applications. In the winter, when environmental factors tend to dry out the skin, be sure to use a moisturizer that affords better protection.

As you age, the skin around your eyes becomes increasingly thin and delicate and requires special care. This skin has virtually no oil glands, so it needs extra protection and hydration to ward off the signs of aging. You don't necessarily need to apply a special eye cream on this area, but if you use your regular moisturizer, it must be gentle and contain no irritating ingredients. Be careful when putting cream on this area. Gently pat it on and take care not to pull or drag the skin.

If your eyes are puffy, try brewing a cup of strong tea, let it cool, and put a piece of tissue soaked in the cool tea under each eye. Another method to reduce puffiness is to hold an ice-cold spoon (place it in the freezer for a couple of minutes first) to the skin under the eyes.

MOISTURIZER BELLS AND WHISTLES

The best moisturizers work because they are a well-balanced formulation of several different hydrating agents. Cosmetics companies are constantly trying to develop new and improved products. Here is a guide to some of the more common bells and whistles added to moisturizers.

Ceramides. Ceramides are a type of lipid and a common ingredient used in moisturizers that seek to stimulate barrier repair. As you will recall, the protective membrane of the stratum corneum is composed of flattened corneocytes. These are glued together by ceramides and other fats, such as cholesterol and free fatty acids, forming a highly effective shield against moisture loss. Ceramides are also capable of binding water molecules, facilitating

---

TABLE 7.6

Moisturizers Suitable for Maturing Skin

- Pond's Nourishing Moisturizer SPF 15
- Almay Moisture Balance Moisture Lotion SPF 15
- Clinique Dramatically Different Moisturizing Lotion
- Estée Lauder Future Perfect Micro-targeted Skin Gel
- Clarins Extra-Firming Day Cream
- L'Oréal Plenitude Hydra-Renewal
- Cetaphil Moisturizing Cream
- Oil of Olay Sensitive Skin Replenishing Cream
- Nutraderm (for dry and sensitive skin)

---

the movement of water into the skin. Under normal conditions, they make up 40 to 65 percent of the lipids of the skin, and they are key to the skin's natural water-regulating capacity.

In an effort to duplicate the effects of the skin's own ceramides, some moisturizers contain ceramides (or their chemical precursor, cerebrosides), derived from animal nervous system tissue. Topical application of ceramides is thought to improve the skin's water retention and to help restore the barrier function of dry skin, increasing its ability to retain moisture and improving its structure and texture. However, the studies on which these claims are based are somewhat preliminary.

Collagen. The notion that you can strengthen the skin's collagen structure by applying a collagen-containing cream is certainly appealing. Unfortunately, when it comes to matters of the human body, things are rarely that simple. Collagen molecules are very large and are unable to penetrate the outer layers of the skin and migrate into the collagen structure in the dermis. Even when collagen is supplied directly by injecting it into the dermis (see chapter 11), it is not incorporated into the skin's permanent collagen structure; it only plumps up the skin temporarily.

While collagen as a cosmetic ingredient has little impact on the skin's natural collagen content, it does afford some benefit when present in a moisturizer. Collagen functions a bit like an emollient, filling in fine cracks and unevenness on the skin's surface and creating a thin, moisture-sealing film on the surface of the skin. The same is true for *elastin,* another natural skin component, which is sometimes included in moisturizers. It cannot be absorbed into the skin, but it can help lock in moisture and smooth out surface irregularities.

Cosmetic Natural Moisturizing Factor. Some the substances that form the skin's natural moisturizing factor are often added to moisturizers to replicate the effect of the NMF on the skin. Urea, for example, is a common moisturizer additive with humectant properties. It diffuses easily into the outer layers of the stratum corneum and considerably enhances its water-holding capacity. Other NMF agents contained in moisturizers include pyrrolidone carboxylic acid (PCA), propylene glycol, lactic acid, and amino acids. While these substances do increase the water-binding properties of moisturizers, they can cause irritation when added in too large quantities. Formulating a moisturizer that combines a high degree of effectiveness with optimum skin friendliness is no simple task.

Hyaluronic acid. Some moisturizers give top billing to hyaluronic acid, one of the glycosaminoglycans (GAGs), the skin's own water-absorbing proteins. The hyaluronic acid content of the skin declines with age, and by the time you reach fifty, your skin contains about half the hyaluronic acid it did when you were younger.

As in the case of collagen, it is appealing to imagine that the decline in hyaluronic acid can be counteracted by applying it topically via moisturizing creams or lotions. However, while hyaluronic acid can serve a useful purpose as a water-binding agent in a well-formulated moisturizer, it will not perform any anti-aging miracles on your skin.

Delivery Systems: Liposomes and Microsponges. Cosmetic chemists have little difficulty loading up a moisturizer with skin-friendly nutrients and hydrating agents. Making sure they retain their potency and actually reach the target tissue is an entirely different matter, however. The stratum corneum is a tightly packed membrane, designed to keep foreign substances out, no matter how beneficial they might be to the deeper layers of skin tissue. Furthermore, many potentially useful skin nutrients are highly volatile and may lose their potency before they reach the target tissue, or they may interact with other ingredients in the formulation and lose their effectiveness. Last, some agents work better if they are released over time, rather than all at once at the time of application.

As a consequence, much effort is put into developing various types of delivery systems that will enhance the effectiveness of certain ingredients. One attempt to address this dilemma, liposomes, are microscopic sacs or spheres with a lipid membrane designed to transport active ingredients inside the sac to the skin. (Fat-soluble compounds penetrate the stratum corneum more easily.) Liposomes can also slow the release of certain compounds, such as vitamin A, so that skin metabolism can keep up with the rate of release.

An alternate delivery system is to use microsponges and polypores (listed in the ingredients as "alkyl methacrylates crosspolymer"). These delivery vehicles similarly encapsulate unstable or irritating agents. Rather than being microscopic "containers," they are tiny sponges that release their content slowly with pressure or heat from the skin.

There are many different types of delivery systems, and products using them often make exaggerated claims. Research in this area is still in its infancy, and there is no guarantee yet that liposomes perform the functions they are thought to. It pays to do a bit of research to see if the promises can be substantiated. Call the manufacturer to find out details about what type of targeted delivery system is used, what the target is, and what research evidence the company has that the delivery actually takes place.

While moisturizers serve a useful function in keeping the skin hydrated and curbing the appearance of fine lines on dry skin, their effect tends to disappear as soon as the moisturizer wears off or is washed off. This is not to say that moisturizers should not be a component of your skin care repertoire—for people with dry skin, they are absolutely essential. However, once you get to the other side of thirty (or before, if you are really serious about anti-aging skin care), it is time to start incorporating some of the treatments that are known to slow the onslaught of aging.

There are several products on the market that can curb intrinsic aging and even reverse some of the damage wrought by extrinsic aging, including photodamage. In the following chapter, we take a look at how you can use these to take greater control of your long-term appearance—in the comfort of your own home and without going to great expense.

CHAPTER 8

Age-Defying Home Care Treatments

*F*or someone age forty-seven, Ivonna's skin was quite well preserved, with fine lines around the eyes and mouth, but no deep wrinkles. Still, though she clearly had been a beauty in her younger days, her appearance was marred by early signs of photoaging. Her skin was sallow and leathery, and an unflattering, blotchy pigmentation on her cheeks gave her face an uneven, mottled tone.

"I thought these were just oversized freckles and something I had to live with," Ivonna explained, referring to the blotchy spots on her cheeks. "But one of my friends says it's sun damage, and that it can be treated."

Ivonna's friend was right. The oversized, blotchy "freckles" were a mild form of melasma, a dyspigmentation that often develops in pregnant women, but that is also a common reaction to photodamage. In addition, the large pores in Ivonna's forehead and her rough skin texture spoke volumes about long hours spent in the sun.

Ivonna was sent home with a prescription for Renova, a cream containing the vitamin-A derivative, tretinoin, which has proven to be effective at reversing some signs of photoaging. Like many women, Ivonna had known about Renova (and its cousin, Retin-A), but had hesitated to use it, because she was fearful of the redness and flaky skin it sometimes creates. However, once she heard that the risk of such reactions was much smaller if she started gradually with a low-concentration cream, she was willing to give it a try.

In the beginning, she noticed some enhanced skin sensitivity and flakiness around her mouth, so she applied the product only every other day. After a couple of weeks, the sensitivity subsided, and she was able to move on to daily use without any adverse effects.

Within three months, she reported that she was thrilled with the results. The brown spots were clearly fading, and her skin texture was smoother and firmer. Some of the crow's-feet around her eyes also appeared to be diminished. Best of all, her skin was less sallow, and a healthy, rosy glow was returning to her face. Ivonna was elated . . . and astounded.

"All these years I've been trying so many different kinds of products, and I've never seen much of a difference," she declared at a follow-up visit. "I can't believe something actually works!"

Ivonna is not unusual. There are several topical treatments available today that can limit or improve age-related skin damage. Unfortunately, so many new and sensational "miracle" products are constantly clamoring for women's attention that it can be hard to discern what works and what doesn't. Many women move from one product to the next in a restless search for the final answer to their skin care woes. This is unfortunate, because it takes staying power to derive benefits from the products that do work. Most skin care products need to be used consistently over a six- to twelve-month period to exert their full effects. More information is needed, so women won't waste their time and money on products of dubious merit.

A Revolution in the Making?

An exciting, new generation of skin care treatments is emerging, which afford therapeutic benefits that can effect permanent changes to the skin's structure and texture. This development is so significant that we may be standing at the threshold of a true revolution in skin care.

These new, age-defying products are a hybrid of cosmetics and pharmaceuticals, which has earned them the name *cosmeceuticals*. Cosmeceuticals contain substances that are pharmacologically active, that is, they have specific therapeutic effects on the skin. As such, they come very close to the definition of drugs, which are substances that can alter the structure or function of human tissue to prevent or treat disease. While standard moisturizers create temporary results, cosmeceuticals include ingredients that create permanent results by modifying the skin's underlying structure.

You will never see cosmetics ads proclaiming that a skin care product has therapeutic properties. That would classify the product as a drug and subject it to much more stringent FDA regulation. Nonetheless, more and more products are aiming to work at the deeper layers of the skin to afford permanent beneficial changes. Most cosmeceuticals have remained classified as "cosmetics" by the FDA, even though they act on human tissue, because they are intended to affect appearance rather than treat disease. Nonetheless, to keep this privilege, cosmetic companies are careful to phrase their product claims so that no direct therapeutic effects are implied.

The cosmeceuticals boom started in the early 1990s with the introduction of alpha hydroxy acids (AHAs). Since then, cosmeceuticals have developed into one of the fastest-growing segments of the cosmetics market, growing at a rate of 15 to 18 percent per year. Products containing AHAs, vitamins and antioxidants, and numerous botanical substances are flooding the market, claiming scientifically verified benefits and clamoring for women's attention.

While you can find much that is beneficial in the emerging science of cosmeceuticals, you also need to do your homework. Some cosmeceuticals really can reduce wrinkles and reverse photoaging, and their benefits are well-documented. Others show promise, but they still have far to go before their benefits for the skin are firmly established. It is important to understand the differences in the benefits various products confer, how to use different types of products, and how to minimize any drawbacks associated with regular use.

Smoothing Fine Lines and Enhancing Skin Texture: AHAs and BHAs

The arrival of alpha hydroxy and beta hydroxy acids (BHAs) on the skin care scene in the early 1990s was hailed as a sensational breakthrough. In truth, however, most good things have been around before, and AHAs are no exception. Foods with natural acidic ingredients have been used to exfoliate the skin since Cleopatra took her first bath in sour milk (the lactic acid in milk has exfoliating properties). The noblewomen at the French court of Louis XIV were famous for pampering their faces with wine (wine contains tartaric acid, another exfoliant). The newer, chemically isolated versions of AHAs and BHAs do the same thing, only in a more scientific application.

As their names imply, alpha hydroxy acids and beta hydroxy acids are mild acids that strip off the top layers of skin. They work primarily by accelerating cell turnover. When you remove the dead cells in the outer layer of the skin, the younger and healthier cells underneath rise to the surface more quickly.

AHAs can perform wonders on photoaged skin. Acidic exfoliation balances irregular skin tones and makes the skin appear fresher and smoother, with a more youthful and healthier glow. Regular use of exfoliants thickens the skin and reduces skin sagging. There is also evidence that such use boosts collagen production and reduces sign of photoaging, such as fine lines, leathery texture, and skin discoloration (particularly when used with a skin lightener, such as hydroquinone). AHAs and BHAs even enhance skin hydration, because they draw water from deeper levels of the skin, giving the skin a plumper and younger look.

The most commonly used AHAs are lactic acid (derived from milk) and glycolic acid (derived from honey or sugarcane). Other AHAs include malic acid from apples and pears, citric acid from lemons and oranges, and tartaric acid from fermented grapes. Glycolic acid is the most thoroughly researched AHA, and there is evidence that it penetrates the skin's outer layers more effectively than other AHAs. The most commonly used BHA is salicylic acid, derived from willow bark. Salicylic acid is also a staple ingredient in many acne products.

In studies testing different concentrations of AHAs, dermatologists have found that products with weaker concentrations, such as 5 percent lactic acid, faciliate skin turnover and increase the smoothness and texture of the epidermis. With a 12 percent solution, changes are found at the level of the dermis as well. Products with a 20 percent concentration increase collagen gene expression and skin content of hyaluronic acid over a three-month period. In stronger concentrations of 30 to 70 percent, alpha hydroxy acids are used by cosmetologists and dermatologists as chemical peels to treat advanced photoaging. At this strength, there are risks of complications such as burns and other skin reactions, so if you do choose this type of treatment, do it under a doctor's supervision. (See chapter 10 for more about using chemical peels to treat photoaging.)

The exfoliating properties of BHAs are not as well researched as those of glycolic acid and lactic acid. However, BHAs are thought to have deeper action because they are fat-soluble and can penetrate deeper into the pores. Products based on this hydroxy acid generally have a lower concentration of 1 to 2 percent, and they are sometimes recommended for people with sensitive skin.

Exfoliating products are big business, but unfortunately, not all products on the market are equally effective. Unless a product lists the percentage of AHAs contained in it, chances are that it has too little to make a difference. You need at least 4 percent AHAs to derive benefits, but by some estimates, the average over-the-counter (OTC) cream contains only about 3 percent AHAs. In addition, the product must have a pH value of between 3 and 5 to have an effect. If the pH value is too high (too alkaline), the exfoliating acids are neutralized; if the pH is too low (too acidic), the product will sting and irritate the skin. You can test a product's pH value using nitrozine test strips available at drugstores.

Don't rush out and buy a product with the strongest concentration of AHAs you can find. AHAs can cause irritation, particularly on sensitive skin, and the higher the concentration, the greater the risk. Start with lower concentrations and work your way up. Prolonged skin irritation can cause a breakdown of the skin tissue, which can translate into faster skin aging and increased wrinkles. If you have sensitive skin, even lower concentrations of AHAs may not be suitable for you.

The long-term effects of using AHAs in high concentrations are unknown. The FDA is currently studying this, but the results won't be out for several years. What we do know is that exfoliating products increase the skin's sensitivity to the sun, predisposing you to more sun damage and photoaging. This risk can be controlled if you are diligent about using sunscreen. The increased sensitivity disappears a week after you stop using an

AHA Products with Known Concentrations

- *The Alpha Hydrox line.* Offers reasonably priced moisturizers with AHA concentrations from 5 to 10 percent. Available in many drugstores or from Neoteric Cosmetics at www.alphahydrox.com or 1-800-447-1919.
- *Aqua Glycolic Face Cream with 10 percent glycolic acid.* Available from Merz Pharmaceuticals at www.aquaglycolic.com or 1-800-253-9499.
- *Neostrata Skin Smoothing creams and lotions, 8–10 percent.* See www.neostrata.com or call 1-800-628-9904.

For AHA products with high concentrations, check out:

- *M.D. Formulations.* Offers glycolic acid compounds with concentrations of 10–15 percent; see www.mdformulations.com or 1-800-MDformula.
- *M.D. Forté.* Contains buffered glycolic acid compounds available in strengths of 12–30 percent. Available through physicians; see www.allergan.com or 800-377-7790.

AHA product, so if you're planning a vacation in the sun, discontinue using AHA products a week before you leave and don't resume treatment until you're back.

According to the Cosmetic, Toiletry and Fragrance Association, AHAs are safe for home use in concentrations of 10 percent or less. (For sensitive skin, a 5 percent concentration is typically the recommended maximum.) Start with a single daily application of a product with an AHA concentration of 7 to 8 percent. Gently apply a pea-sized amount to your face in the evening after cleansing your skin.

If your skin becomes flaky, dry, pink, or sore, cut down use to every other day or twice a week, or try a lower concentration. You can also try a product with buffered glycolic acid, which is less acidic and better tolerated by the skin.

If you don't develop any problems, you can move on to products with a 10 percent concentration or to twice-daily applications after four to five weeks. Little is known about the effects of long-term use of AHA products with a 15 to 20 percent concentration, so if you want to use stronger products, limit use to once or twice a month.

Physicians often recommend that to avoid undue irritation, regular applications after the first six months should be cycled, two or three months on, two or three months off, to allow the skin to rest. Alternatively, you can simply cut down your use to every other day after the first six months and see if that is enough to retain the results. Once you start using AHA products, never, ever venture outside (in any kind of weather) without wearing a sunscreen with at least an SPF 15.

The Bottom Line. Chemical exfoliators are among the few cosmetic substances whose claim to fame is based on extensive research. They treat fine lines, improve skin texture, and create a more even and youthful complexion in almost every age group. If your skin can tolerate it, a good AHA or BHA product should be an essential part of your anti-aging arsenal. People in their seventies and older should not use this type of product, as it would harm their delicate skin.

Erasing Wrinkles with the Retinoids

For skin care that packs a more powerful age-defying punch, a trip to your dermatologist is worth your while. He or she can give you a prescription for products that have the capacity to reverse both intrinsic and extrinsic aging of the skin.

We are talking, of course, about skin care products containing the vitamin A derivatives known as *retinoids*. While vitamin A in the food you eat is important for skin health and renewal in general, topical application of certain vitamin A derivatives has specific and important anti-aging effects. In particular, one member of the retinoid family known as *tretinoin* (short for all-trans-retinoic acid) has proven to be effective in treating photoaged and wrinkled skin. Tretinoin is the active ingredient in products such as Retin-A and Renova, two of the most well-known and well-researched anti-aging treatments around. Tretinoin is classified as a drug, because it was pioneered as a disease treatment and alters the function and structure of the skin, so you need a prescription for tretinoin-based products.

Retin-A was first developed and tested in the 1970s for treating acne. Dermatologists noticed that, over a period of time, the skin of acne patients using Retin-A began to look younger and took on a rosier glow, had improved texture, and fewer lines and freckles. Needless to say, word got out quickly, and by the late 1980s, Retin-A had gained a widespread reputation as a miracle cure for aging skin. In 1995, Ortho Dermatological, the manufacturer of Retin-A, introduced a more skin-friendly version of Retin-A called Renova. Renova (0.02 percent or 0.05 percent tretinoin) is formulated as a

Spotlight on Research

THE BENEFITS OF TRETINOIN

Key research findings for tretinoin-based creams include:

- increased blood flow, collagen formation, and GAG content in elderly skin;
- restored collagen formation in photoaged skin over a ten- to twelve-month period;
- disappearance of fine wrinkles and improved skin color and texture after four months; and
- alleviation of coarse wrinkling and improved pigmentation after six months.

Naturally, results differ from person to person and depend on the concentration used and frequency of application.

rich moisturizer, which helps counteract the drying effect of tretinoin. Renova was the first skin care product to gain FDA approval for treating photodamaged and wrinkled skin.

Today, several forms of tretinoin cream are available. They all contain the same active ingredient, but differ in concentration and in the type of vehicle they use to deliver tretinoin to the skin. Avita® (0.025 percent tretinoin), available in a cream or gel, is designed to release tretinoin slowly onto the skin. Retin-A Micro® (0.04 percent or 0.1 percent tretinoin) uses microsponge technology, which also releases the active ingredient more slowly and hence causes less irritation to the skin. Both are typically used to treat acne in people with sensitive skin. If you want to treat wrinkles but are prone to acne, these formulations are your best bet.

Regular use of tretinoin-based products reverses intrinsic and extrinsic aging. Tretinoin exfoliates the skin as AHAs and BHAs do, causing faster cell turnover, but at a deeper level. It stimulates the growth of new blood vessels, which leads to improved circulation and enhances production of collagen, giving the skin a firmer texture. Studies have shown that long-term use of a tretinoin-based cream makes the top layer of the skin thicker and more compact and reduces pore size, making the skin smoother. Unsightly age spots, caused by excessive or uneven deposits of melanin, are sloughed off with the top layers of skin. Best of all, wrinkles caused by sun damage are reduced in both number and depth.

The effectiveness of tretinoin-based products depends on the concentration and the length of the treatment. Dermatologists have long thought that concentrations of 0.1 percent were the most effective for treating photoaging. However, recent evidence shows that considerable results can be achieved at concentrations as low as 0.025 percent. This is good news, because the lower the tretinoin concentration, the less the product will irritate the skin.

A fairly high percentage of people using tretinoin-based products develop a "retinoid reaction," which shows up as redness, dryness, flaky skin, and a burning sensation. People with skin types I and II usually exhibit greater sensitivity to tretinoin, as do people with cosmetic allergies, very dry skin, or with skin problems such as eczema and rosacea. People with fair and dry skin typically do not tolerate concentrations above 0.05 percent very well. People with darker skin or with advanced photodamage have better tolerance and can often move on to a 0.1 percent tretinoin cream after three to four months.

The correct concentration for you is the one your skin can tolerate every night without any visible reactions. If you develop redness or flaky skin, reduce the strength of the cream you use or apply the product less frequently until the reaction subsides.

Ask the Doctor

Q. *There are many over-the-counter products containing vitamin A derivatives that sound like they do much the same job as Renova and Retin-A. Why should I go through all the trouble of getting a prescription for a tretinoin-based product?*

A. Like you, many women hesitate to see a dermatologist just to get a prescription for a skin care product. Cosmetics companies know that, and they have been quick to introduce products with ingredients that sound like they offer much the same benefits.

There are many forms of retinoids; tretinoin just happens to be the one with the best-documented topical benefits. Other retinoids, such as *retinol, retinyl,* and *retinyl palmitate* have become popular ingredients in numerous moisturizers claiming similar antiwrinkle effects.

Unfortunately, while many of these products are less irritating to the skin, they are not as chemically active and effective as tretinoin. Retinol (pure vitamin A) is unstable and loses potency over time. In addition, it takes more retinol than tretinoin to produce results. There is some evidence that a 1 percent solution of retinol produces results; however, at these concentrations, retinol irritates the skin. To avoid this, most companies include too little retinol—as little as 0.1 percent—in their products to have much effect.

For the other retinoid derivatives, such as retinyl palmitate and retinyl linoleate, the news is no more encouraging. Retinyl palmitate, for example, is only half as strong as retinol, and while it may alleviate dry skin, it has no documented effects on wrinkles.

Start applying a thin layer of the cream every other night for the first few weeks until your skin adapts, then increase to every night. (Day use is not advised, because tretinoin is chemically affected by sunlight.) Apply a pea-sized amount to your face at night after cleaning and drying your face. Make sure your face is completely dry before applying the cream. In the morning, remove the cream by washing your face thoroughly, but don't scrub or rub.

Tretinoin creams dry the skin and should always be used with a gentle moisturizer. Apply the moisturizer in the morning after you wash your face and as often as needed during the day. In addition, since tretinoin creams increase the skin's sensitivity to sunlight, it is essential that you use a sunscreen of at least SPF 15 whenever you venture out. Wear a hat and, as much as possible, avoid exposure to direct sunlight.

Although results vary, the effects often become visible rather quickly. Within a month, you will probably feel that your skin is smoother. After three months of regular use, it is common to see a reduction in wrinkles and a lightening of age spots or freckles. Oddly, some people don't respond at all to tretinoin. If you use the cream regularly and don't see any improvement within four months, it is unlikely that your skin will respond.

It takes eight to twelve months of regular use for the effects to peak. After that, you can reduce use to two to three times a week. This type of maintenance therapy is necessary; to retain results, you will need to use the cream for the rest of your life.

Do not use tretinoin-based creams if you are planning to become pregnant or if you are pregnant or breastfeeding. People who are photosensitive or who take medications that cause photosensitivity also should not use this type of remedy. Use of these creams should always be under the supervision of a doctor. If your skin doesn't tolerate Renova well, your doctor might try a different concentration or one of the other types of tretinoin products on the market.

The Bottom Line. No other treatment for photoaging has benefits as thoroughly documented as tretinoin. The treatment is simple and easy to incorporate into your daily skin care routine. Unless your skin is sensitive, adverse reactions often can be avoided by starting slowly and giving your skin plenty of time to adapt. Begin by applying the product every other day, and then work your way up to greater frequency. Although it is always preferable to consult with a dermatologist in person, many websites now offer Renova and Retin-A by way of an online doctor's consultation. Direct contact with your physician is always preferable.

KINETIN (FURFURYLADENINE)

Kinetin, or *N6-furfuryladenine*, is a plant growth hormone that exerts important anti-aging effects in plants, such as slowing the yellowing of leaves and degeneration of fruits. Kinetin also has been shown to extend the average life span of fruit flies when it is added to their diet.

Most of the published research on kinetin concerns its effects in plant systems. Research on its action in more complex biological systems, such as mammalian animals and humans, is considerably more sparse. Preliminary evidence indicates that when kinetin is added to a medium containing human skin fibroblasts, it delays the onset of numerous cellular changes associated with aging. These research results also suggest that kinetin may be even more effective in preventing age-related changes than in reversing existing age-induced deterioration.

When it comes to the actual effects of applying kinetin to human skin, the research is quite limited. The few clinical studies available are sponsored by Senetek PLC, the company that holds the rights to the patents on kinetin. While studies by independent researchers are needed to develop a broader picture on the effects of kinetin, early evidence shows promise. Studies have found that twice-daily application of kinetin produces improvements on several markers of photodamage, including fine and coarse wrinkles, mottled pigmentation, skin roughness, and fine spider veins. Even more significant, these effects developed without the typical negative side effects of AHA and tretinoin use, such as stinging, redness, increased dryness or peeling, and general skin irritation. Kinetin also improved moisture retention by strengthening the skin's natural barrier function.

A limited number of companies have received licenses to produce skin care products containing kinetin. These include the Body Shop (Skin Re-Leaf with Kinetin), ICN Pharmaceuticals (Kinerase®, with 0.1% kinetin), Osmotics (Osmotics Kinetin skin care line), and Revlon (Almay Kinetine skin care line).

The Bottom Line. Early research evidence indicates that kinetin may benefit photodamaged skin, without the skin irritation produced by tretinoin and AHAs. However, the research is still too limited to draw firm conclusions. Nonetheless, products containing kinetin may be worth a try, particularly if your skin is sensitive and you don't tolerate tretinoin-based or AHA products very well. Look for products containing a 0.1 percent concentration of kinetin.

Skin Antioxidants— A Skin Care Revolution in the Making?

The effects of topical applications of tretinoin are noteworthy for more than their anti-aging benefits. They demonstrate that a skin-friendly nutrient, in this case a derivative of vitamin A, also has benefits when applied topically.

Might other vitamins or nutrients that support skin health have similar benefits if applied directly to the skin? In particular, since free radical damage is known to be a major factor in skin aging, could antioxidants applied directly to the skin prevent or reverse such damage?

This thinking has become the leading premise behind one of the hottest new trends in skin care. The number of products containing vitamins has more than tripled over the last ten years, and new products are constantly emerging. While many offerings in this mushrooming category of skin care products show promise, scientific research documenting their effects often lags behind. In many cases, it is too early to tell which agents will live up to their promises; however, this is an extremely exciting and promising field of research and definitely worth a closer look.

VITAMIN C

One of the major antioxidant vitamins, vitamin C, is essential for collagen formation and skin renewal. Unfortunately, only an estimated 8 percent of the vitamin C you eat ever makes it to your skin. This makes a persuasive case for applying it directly to the skin, where higher doses might trigger significant anti-aging benefits.

Research on the effects of topical application of vitamin C is of relatively recent origin, but results have been promising. There is some evidence that vitamin C (alone or combined with vitamin E) might protect against sun damage when it is applied directly to the skin, possibly by increasing the skin's antioxidant reserves.

Other studies indicate that topical use of vitamin C might actually *reverse* photodamage. One double-blind study found a significant decrease in wrinkling and improved hydration on the area of the face treated with vitamin C over a twelve-week period. The study used a formulation with both a water-soluble and a fat-soluble form of vitamin C (10 percent ascorbic acid and 7 percent tretrahexyldecyl ascorbate). Another study using L-ascorbic acid also resulted in reduced wrinkling, smoother skin, and better skin tone and color.

Topical application of vitamin C has also been found to stimulate collagen production and improve skin texture and firmness

Vitamin C Products

Products containing L-ascorbic acid in concentrations of 10 to 15 percent:

- Cellex-C®. One of the more well-researched vitamin C products. Products contain 10–17.5 percent ascorbic acid along with zinc and the amino acid tyrosine, both of which are said to further facilitate skin remodeling and repair; see www. cellexc.com or call 1-800-Cellex-C.
- Complex-C™. Contains 10 percent ascorbic acid along with retinol; see www.complexc.com or call 1-866-475-4424.
- Citrix-C Cream with 10–15 percent asorbic acid. See www.clavin.com/clavin_labs/p_vitamin_c.htm or call 1-888-372-5284.
- Skinceuticals Topical Vitamin-C, Serum 10 or Serum 15. Contains ascorbic acid in concentrations of 10 or 15 percent; see www.skinceuticals.com or call 1-800-811-1660.
- EmerginC Vitamin C Serum or Cream. Products contain two forms of vitamin C, L-ascorbic acid and magnesium ascorbyl phosphate. Many are formulated with additional agents to enhance antioxidant protection or reduce skin irritation; see www.emerginc.com or call 1-800-257-9597.

Products containing ascorbyl palmitate:

- Vitamin C Ester Concentrated Restorative Cream with DMAE or Vitamin C Amine Complex Face Lift with DMAE. Developed by Dr. Nicholas Perricone, the leading advocate of the anti-aging benefits of vitamin C ester; see www.clinicalcreations.com or call 1-888-823-7837.
- Alpha Lipoic Acid, Vitamin C Ester, and Dimethylaminoetranol (DMAE) Cream. See www.revivalabs.com or call 1-800-257-7774, ext. 19.

in postmenopausal women. The improvement was largest in the women who ingested the least amount of vitamin C through their daily diet.

While such research is promising, many questions still need to be addressed. Studies are typically done under ideal conditions, meaning that researchers make sure the type of vitamin C used retains maximum potency and is applied in sufficient concentrations to produce an effect. In real life, unfortunately, it is not that simple. Vitamin C needs to be present in an active concentration of at least 5 percent to have any benefits, yet most forms of vitamin C are very unstable. A product might have the right potency when it leaves the manufacturing plant but lose it by the time it is applied to your skin. Furthermore, high concentrations of vitamin C cause skin irritation in some people, so there are limits to how potent the products can be.

Most important, it is still unclear which forms of vitamin C are most suitable for cosmetic uses. L-ascorbic acid is used in a number of products, but for maximum potency, it must be present in concentrations of at least 10 percent and embedded in formulations with a pH level of less than 3.5. This greatly increases the risk of skin irritation, particularly if you are also using AHAs or Renova.

Another form of vitamin C, vitamin C ester (ascorbyl palmitate) emerged recently as an anti-aging contender. There is some evidence that topical application of this type of vitamin C can protect against sun-induced redness and inflammation in human skin. However, the results are preliminary, and few studies have been conducted by independent researchers on the effects of this type of vitamin C.

The Bottom Line. The most thoroughly researched form of vitamin C is L-ascorbic acid in concentrations of 5 to 15 percent. L-ascorbic acid has been found to improve photodamaged skin in several studies. Products containing L-asorbic acids in these concentrations may have a very low pH value, meaning that they are

The Informed Consumer

WHEN IS RESEARCH RESEARCH?
Scientific research is the gold standard by which the effectiveness of any type of product or drug can be determined. When it comes to cosmetic ingredients, however, there is research, and then there is research.

Scientific studies come in many forms. The most reliable information is derived from double-blind, clinical studies performed on humans. In this type of study, participants are assigned randomly to a treatment group, which receives the drug or treatment to be tested, and a control group, which receives a placebo, that is, an inert treatment substitute. A study is double-blind when neither the study participants nor the researchers know who receives which treatment until after the study is completed. (In testing dermatological products and treatments, different skin sites on the same person are often used to test the difference between the active substance and the placebo.) At the end of the test period, the results are analyzed to see if the treatment produced any statistically significant effects.

The quality of a study is often indicated by where it is published. Studies published in peer-reviewed journals have been subjected to rigorous analysis by independent researchers before being accepted for publication.

Because skin care products are not subject to the same stringent FDA regulations as pharmaceuticals, they can be manufactured and sold with little or no testing to verify their effectiveness. Even when testing is done, it is often not done by independent researchers, but rather by the manufacturer of the product or by an agency it hires. Such tests often do not use the same stringent scientific standards, and they are not submitted for publication in peer-reviewed scientific journals and subjected to the rigorous standards of quality control this entails. Unpublished research can be of poor quality, biased, and of little scientific merit. Similarly, the results of studies performed on animals or cell cultures in a laboratory dish (the technical term is *in vitro*) should be regarded as tentative.

When an ad for a skin care product claims that the product is "clinically proven to ..." or "laboratory tested" or "dermatologist tested," look to see if the ad references a published study using human subjects (or call the company to ask for a reference). If there is no such reference, the claims may mean little or nothing.

very acidic and could irritate the skin, particularly if it is dry and sensitive. Apply them only once a day and don't use vitamin C products along with other types of cosmeceuticals known to cause skin irritation, such as AHAs and Retin-A or Renova.

VITAMIN E

Several studies indicate that vitamin E (as alpha-tocopherol) protects against UV-induced oxidative damage when applied directly to the skin. Vitamin E is thought to exert this effect by increasing the skin's antioxidant reserves and by absorbing ultraviolet radiation. When used in combination with vitamin C, vitamin E increases the protective effects of sunscreen. It has also been shown to reduce certain types of photodamage to the DNA that can be precursors to skin cancer. The greater the dose of vitamin E applied to the skin, the greater the protection afforded.

The specific anti-aging effects of topical vitamin E on human skin are not as thoroughly researched as those of vitamin C, but early results show promise. Vitamin E has been shown to reduce skin wrinkling in hairless mice (an animal often used in experiments, because its skin reacts similarly to human skin). In vitro studies (using human cell cultures in lab dishes) indicate that it might protect collagen from free radical damage.

While all four forms of vitamin E (as tocopherol) have protective benefits, some studies suggest that topical applications of alpha-tocopherol might be five to ten times as effective as other forms of vitamin E. The type of vitamin E most commonly added to skin care products, alpha-tocopherol acetate, appears to provide less protection.

While the jury is still out on its age-defying virtues, vitamin E does have several known benefits. Included in a skin care product (as tocopherol), vitamin E helps to preserve the fatty components in cosmetic creams. It is often used in moisturizers and other skin care products as an emollient, because it softens and

Spotlight on Research:

CAN SUPPLEMENTS PROTECT AGAINST PHOTODAMAGE?

Topical application of antioxidant vitamins C and E can protect against sunburn and long-term photo-damage; however, much the same effect can be obtained by taking these vitamins in supplement form. Some studies have shown that people supplementing their daily diet with vitamin C (2,000 mg ascorbic acid) and vitamin E (1,000 IU of d-alpha-tocopherol) become more resistant to sunburn after only eight days. Similar results have been found in individuals taking a mixture of antioxidant substances, including vitamins C and E, carotenoids, selenium, and proanthocyanidins.

smoothes the skin and helps increase moisture content. When added to sunscreens, vitamin E can enhance the product's effectiveness, but look for suncreens containing the alpha-tocopherol form of the vitamin.

The Bottom Line. Vitamin E holds some promise for anti-aging skin care, but the research is still limited, and it is too early to draw conclusions. We know very little about which types and concentrations of vitamin E might provide anti-aging benefits. At this point, it's anybody's guess whether any commercial vitamin E creams contain enough of the vitamins to make a difference.

COENZYME Q10

Coenzyme Q10 (ubiquinone) or CoQ10 is involved in cellular energy production. It is also a powerful antioxidant that protects the cells from oxidative stress. When taken as a supplement,

The Informed Consumer

COSMETIC CHALLENGES

Manufacturers face numerous obstacles when trying to develop skin care products that use vitamins and other nutrients to improve the skin. Here are some of the questions cosmetic chemists have to tackle:

Does it penetrate the skin? Many potentially nourishing substances cannot penetrate the stratum corneum, which, after all, was created as a barrier to keep out foreign substances. Penetration enhancers can remedy this to some extent, but delivering active ingredients to the deeper levels of the skin is still an issue.

Does it work in topical form? Just because a vitamin or antioxidant exerts benefits when ingested, it won't necessarily have the same effects when it is applied directly to the skin. We still know precious little about the biological mechanisms by which nutrient substances might exert topical effects.

Is the active ingredient present in the right potency and is it sufficiently bioavailable? Too little is useless, and too much could be harmful. In addition, many nutrient agents are unstable and may lose their potency over time or when combined with other ingredients. A product that was effective when it left the manufacturer might have lost its potency by the time it reaches your bathroom shelf.

CoQ10 is known to improve heart health, decrease hypertension, and strengthen immune function. It is particularly plentiful in the skin, where it works with vitamin C and E to boost antioxidant defenses.

The rationale for incorporating CoQ10 into skin care products is similar to that of vitamin C and E. We know that oxidative stress caused by UV radiation and other environmental insults plays a key role in skin's aging. Fortifying the skin's antioxidant defenses by applying CoQ10 topically makes sense, particularly because the amount of CoQ10 in the body declines after age thirty-five to forty. The levels of CoQ10 in the skin are also depleted when the skin is exposed to UV light, making another powerful case for external supplementation.

Here again, the research is in its early stages, but the evidence so far is encouraging. As we grow older, skin cells such as the keratinocytes lose some of their natural resistance to UV radiation. Some studies have shown that topical application of CoQ10 increases resistance to UV radiation in these cells, prevents oxidative damage to cellular DNA, and protects against collagen breakdown.

Protection is one thing, but might CoQ10 be able to reverse photodamage? There are some early indications that it might. A few studies have reported reduced wrinkle depth around the eyes (crow's-feet) following long-term topical application of CoQ10.

The Bottom Line. The reasoning for the benefits of CoQ10 on the skin is persuasive, but more research is needed. While there is evidence that CoQ10 increases the antioxidant resistance of the skin, little is known about what is required for a skin care product to duplicate such results. We need to learn more about which concentrations of CoQ10 are required to afford benefits and which carrier characteristics are needed to preserve its potency.

ALPHA-LIPOIC ACID

As contenders for cosmetic fame go, few substances have enjoyed such a rapid rise as alpha-lipoic acid. Alpha-lipoic acid is a relatively new arrival on the anti-aging scene, although scientists have known about the substance since the 1950s.

Alpha lipoic acid is a vitamin-like nutrient. The body is able to generate it, but it is also derived from certain foods, including yeast and liver. Like CoQ10, it is involved in cellular metabolism and energy production, but what really has researchers excited is that alpha-lipoic acid is an extremely versatile and powerful antioxidant. Because it is both water- and fat-soluble, it can fight free radicals in any part of the cell, making it a potent free radical scavenger. Even more noteworthy, scientists believe it has the ability to "recycle" other antioxidants, such as vitamins C and E. Some experts believe that it might be the most powerful antioxidant of all. In addition, alpha-lipoic acid is thought to have anti-inflammatory properties, and it may stimulate collagen production.

There is little research available on the effects of supplementation on actual human beings, and even less on the potential benefits of topical application of alpha-lipoic acid. However, a preliminary study using a 5 percent alpha-lipoic acid cream over a three-month period did find evidence of decreased wrinkles around the mouth and eyes, decreased pore size, and a more healthier, rosier complexion.

The Bottom Line. Although alpha-lipoic acid has been touted as an age-defying wonder child, the research evidence substantiating the effects of topical application is extremely limited. That is not to say the claims are untrue, only that it is too early to tell. If you like to try new things, and money is not an issue, it is worth giving skin care products containing this antioxidant a try.

COPPER PEPTIDES

Copper plays an important role in collagen production and elastin synthesis. Studies have shown that when the level of copper in the cells is increased, collagen production goes up as well. Internally ingested copper is known to play other vital roles for skin health, including stimulating tissue building and skin repair, enhancing the production of GAGs, and functioning as an antioxidant.

While the benefits of internally ingested copper on the skin are established, we still know very little about the effects of applying copper directly to the skin via creams or serums. Copper in its inorganic form can harm the skin, because it promotes free radical production. But when it is made organic through binding to peptides, it is considered to be safe for the skin. We know that copper peptides stimulate wound healing when applied directly to the skin, but very little research is available on whether they confer any anti-aging benefits.

In one study comparing the effects of tretinoin and copper tripeptides in a culture of dermal fibroblasts, tretinoin was found to stimulate the secretion of different fibroblast growth factors, a possible biological pathway for the skin tightening observed with regular use of tretinoin. Similar effects were not observed for copper tripeptides, however. A few industry-sponsored studies have reported that creams containing copper peptides produce some improvement in fine wrinkling, facial pigmentation, and skin thickness. It is unclear, however, whether the improvements were considerable enough to translate into clearly visible results.

The Bottom Line. Like many other cosmeceutical agents, copper shows promise, but more research is needed on its effects on aging skin. On the plus side, creams containing copper are nonirritating and generally less costly than most other cosmeceuticals, which makes them a good choice for budget-oriented consumers.

Putting Together a Daily Skin Rejuvenation Regimen

The importance of antioxidants in maintaining health and combating aging is well documented. While the research on topical antioxidants is in an early phase, antioxidant skin care products are definitely worth a second look. The key to a great skin rejuvenation regimen is to make the most of what science and technology have to offer, even if the results are still tentative.

At the same time, putting together a good daily rejuvenation regime is not about chasing after every new product that promises eternal youth. Rather, it involves zeroing in on the ingredients that work well for your skin and using them long enough to benefit from their full effects. None of the rejuvenation treatments currently available is perfect, but in combination, they can produce significant effects. Here are some guidelines to put together an anti-aging regimen that works for you:

- *Start with the true and tried.* If you have any signs of photoaging (and who doesn't?), you owe it to your skin to give either AHAs or retinoid products (Renova, Retin-A) a try. If you use AHAs, use only products that list the AHA concentration they contain; anything else is a waste of time.
- *Use only a couple of products at a time.* If you use too many products at once, it is hard to determine which ones make a difference. Start with one product to establish a baseline, then add another later. Never layer products; instead, apply them at different times of day.
- *Don't combine products with irritating ingredients.* If you are already using a product known to cause skin irritation, such as one containing AHAs, don't add another, such as products containing vitamin C. (In the case of AHAs and Renova, some skin types do well combining the two treatments, but don't try this without first consulting with your dermatologist.)
- *Think long term.* Skin renewal is a slow process; you need to allow at least six months for results to emerge, and in some cases even longer. And don't stop using a product just because you've attained the results you wanted. Maintenance therapy is essential to retain results.
- *Vary your routine.* Your best bet is to start with products that have been proven to have an effect and then vary your routine over time. In that way, you give yourself a chance to see what works for you.
- *Remember the three basic rules of anti-aging skin care.* SPF 15 . . . SPF 15 . . . SPF 15 . . .

PART IV

Erasing Aging:
Advanced Treatments
For a More Youthful You

CHAPTER 9

New Tools in the Fight Against Aging

*A*t age thirty-five, with perfect, unblemished skin and no beauty concerns to speak of, Carey is not the kind of person you would expect to find in a cosmetic dermatologist's office. Yet Carey has been a regular client of ours since she was thirty-two. She first came in for a consultation because of sun-induced brown spots on her forehead. But she quickly became a regular client once she saw how the treatment we applied also improved her overall complexion and tightened the skin on her forehead and around her eyes.

Carey is part of a new breed of women in their late twenties to mid-forties who are intent on battling wrinkles and other signs of aging before they ever get a chance to emerge. "I figure, if I do what I can to slow aging now," Carey reasons, "I'll benefit through my thirties and forties, and I might just be able to avoid more invasive treatments later."

Carey's observation is insightful, and she is fortunate to be in the right place at the right time. With the increasing popularity of outdoor activities, initial signs of photoaging are becoming apparent in younger and younger individuals, and it is not unusual to see women in their twenties and thirties with early wrinkle formation, pigment changes, and other signs of such damage. But thanks to several recently developed treatment technologies and techniques, there is no longer any need to live with the results of sun damage and other visible signs of aging. In fact, many of these treatments may be just as effective in preventing or slowing development of wrinkles and other signs of aging as they are in removing them. Best of all, these treatments are non-invasive and, for the most part, as effortless and painless as getting a facial. In this chapter, we introduce you to some of the exciting new anti-aging technologies that can help you maintain or restore a youthful appearance.

Photorejuvenation:
A Revolution in Anti-Aging Treatments

The primary antidote to aging skin remains controlling the extrinsic aging factors that we explored in previous chapters. No external treatment, no matter how advanced, can beat the long-term benefits of maintaining a healthy lifestyle, sufficient sun protection, and a daily anti-aging skin care regimen attuned to the specific needs of your skin.

Inevitably, however, sooner or later you have to face the fact that on their own these tools are no longer sufficient to halt the progression of aging. Until very recently, cosmetic surgery was one of the few options available if you wanted to improve your skin after the passage of time had dug "deep trenches in thy beauty's field," as Shakespeare so eloquently put it. These surgical procedures are not only expensive, they are also invasive and often produce less-than-perfect results. Women opting for surgical facelifts, for example, often end up looking gaunt, as if their skin has been stretched and manipulated unnaturally. The intention obviously is to make a person look younger, but the treatment sometimes succeeds only in making her look, well, different. And of course, this kind of surgery involves "going under the knife," which is not a prospect many people find appealing.

Within the past five years, a number of minimally invasive anti-aging treatments have emerged that produce excellent results with little or no downtime and few or no side effects. Often referred to as *photorejuvenation*, these treatments use light energy to rejuvenate the skin. While the term, photorejuvenation, is sometimes used specifically to refer to Intense Pulsed Light™ technology, a type of treatment discussed later, in its broader meaning, the term denotes any treatment used to combat mild to moderate sun-induced aging.

Photorejuvenation is unique because it offers a noninvasive approach to repairing damage to the deeper layers of the skin. Photorejuvenation treatments stimulate the body to produce new collagen to replace damaged parts of the skin. They can reverse such visible signs of sun damage as broken capillaries, dark spots, blotchy skin color, redness of the face and neck, freckles, enlarged pore size, rosacea, and wrinkles.

The Amazing Power of Light: Lasers in Facial Rejuvenation

One of the most significant recent advances in cosmetic dermatology has been the discovery of the many ways laser light can be used to produce facial rejuvenation. The theory of laser light was first laid out by Albert Einstein in 1917, but the first laser was not

Are You a Candidate for Photorejuvenation?

Take the following quiz to determine whether you are a candidate for photorejuvenation and to assess which treatment may be most suitable for you.

POINTS	NO VISIBLE SIGNS 0 PTS.	SOME VISIBLE SIGNS 1 PT.	COULD USE IMPROVE-MENT 2 PTS.	NEEDS IMPROVE-MENT 3 PTS.	NEEDS IMMEDIATE ATTENTION 4 PTS.
REDNESS Broken blood vessels on the face, rosacea, flushing					
PIGMENT DISCOLORATION Brown spots on sun-exposed areas of the skin, also known as "age spots" or "liver spots."					
FINE LINES Fine expression lines that disappear when your face is at rest					
WRINKLES Deep lines that do not disappear when your face is at rest					
POOR SKIN TEXTURE Enlarged pores, coarse-ness, loss of smooth-ness and elasticity					
SUN DAMAGE Uneven, mottled coloration					
OTHER CONCERNS Signs of photodamage on neck, chest, back of hands					

(continued on next page)

Are You a Candidate for Photorejuvenation? (continued)

Add up your points by totaling the numbers associated with each column you have checked.

0–6 points: Your skin is still healthy. Keep up the good work!

7–11 points: Your complexion is starting to show the first signs of sun damage. The noninvasive photorejuvenation treatments described in this chapter will help you reverse some of the damage and prevent further deterioration.

Over 12 points: Your skin is exhibiting significant signs of photo-damage. You will get the best results from the more advanced photorejuvenation procedures described in chapter 10. Once the worst signs of photoaging have improved, the gentle rejuvenating treatments described in this chapter will help you to keep further aging at bay.

Adapted from "Complexion Quiz," Lumenis, Inc.

---

developed until 1960. Since then lasers have become ubiquitous; you find them in everything from supermarket checkout scanners to consumer electronics to the most sophisticated military systems. In medicine, they have found many applications — eye surgery, cardiac surgery, treatment of tumors, surgery of the spine, and so on.

The word, *laser,* is an acronym for Light Amplification by the Stimulated Emission of Radiation. While normal light waves are scattered and incoherent, a laser emits a concentrated, intense beam of one specific wavelength of light. Think of the difference between an army marching in step and a group of people milling around—that's the difference between laser light and normal light. Because of the coherence of the light particles, laser light is so powerful that it is capable of burning through tissue, and it can be aimed in such a precise way that very specific areas of tissue can be targeted. Even in the early days, the technology pointed the way to an entirely new approach to dealing with skin problems. Laser light is able to penetrate and vaporize the thin layers of tissue in the target skin area. It works by creating "controlled damage," then allowing the body's own healing mechanisms to create the desired results, rather than creating an artificial change from the outside.

Laser technology has been greatly refined since early lasers were first introduced in the 1960s. One of the problems with the first lasers used for treating skin conditions was that they were not precise enough. Tissues surrounding the treated area also heated up, increasing the chance of scarring. Over the last decade, however, there has been astonishing progress in laser technology, which has opened up whole new areas for anti-aging skin treatments. Modern lasers are computer-driven, and as computers continue to evolve, so do lasers. Think of the difference between the huge computers in the 1960s that filled an entire room, but had less computing power than the personal computers that began to appear on the market in the 1980s. Then think of how much more sophisticated the laptops we use today are than those early PCs and Macs. The revolution in laser surgery has been just as remarkable, as treatments for skin problems become progressively less and less invasive, with shorter and shorter recovery times.

In line with new technological developments has come new public perception of what laser treatments can do. People have started to realize that lasers are not used solely to treat skin diseases or deformities; they can be used to make you more beautiful and reverse the signs of aging.

Nonablative Facial Resurfacing: The Benefits of "Lunchtime" Lasers

One of the most important uses of lasers in cosmetic dermatology is in facial resurfacing. There are numerous resurfacing treatments, but they all work in the same way. The basic operating principle is the same as for AHAs and BHAs. Essentially, you strip away the outer layers of damaged skin, and as new cells emerge during the healing process, the surface of the skin is transformed and becomes smoother, more youthful, and more evenly pigmented. The difference is largely one of degree. Even the most powerful AHA treatment can only do so much. Lasers can be used for deeper levels of resurfacing, resulting in a deeper level of regeneration and more dramatic results. Laser resurfacing actually rebuilds the skin, erasing old, sun-damaged skin tissue like chalk off a blackboard.

Facial resurfacing has long been the standard tool in the fight against wrinkles and photo damage, but more aggressive treatments, such as deeper chemical peels and standard dermabrasion, are associated with significant discomfort and significant postoperative recovery time. Even the early lasers used for facial resurfacing involved considerable damage to the surface layer of the skin and consequent swelling, redness, bruising, and pain.

In recent years, the no-pain, no-gain school of age-reversing treatments has received serious competition from new high-tech treatments, which literally make reversing the clock as simple and comfortable as having your hair done. This new generation of treatments is *nonablative*, that is, unlike earlier facial resurfacing treatments, these do not remove the surface layer of the skin. As a consequence, if there is pain, it is minimal, there are generally no uncomfortable side effects, and there is no downtime whatsoever.

Nonablative lasers used for facial resurfacing are sometimes popularly known as "lunchtime lasers." Lunchtime lasers are everything anyone ever hoped skin treatments might be: noninvasive, easy, quick, and not too expensive. In fact, they are so quick that you can have one done during your lunch hour and still have time for a sandwich and coffee before heading back to the office.

Best of all, no one will ever know you just underwent a powerful anti-aging treatment, because nonablative treatments do not create a wound in the outer layer of skin. Make no mistake, however; these treatments rejuvenate the skin from the inside out. The results are simple and unmistakable: younger-looking skin, with more collagen and greater elasticity.

There are a number of new lasers used for so-called lunchtime laser treatments, including CoolTouch II®, Smoothbeam™, N-Lite™, and Coolglide® Vantage. The principle behind these new anti-aging treatments is that they minimize the auxiliary tissue damage wrought by the laser's movement over the skin, while retaining many of its beneficial effects. The CoolTouch laser, for example, combines a powerful laser with a cooling cryogen spray. As the laser passes over the skin, the protective cooling spray is applied to the surface of the skin simultaneously, allowing the laser light to pass harmlessly through the upper layer of the skin. The light pulse used with these lasers penetrates to the dermis and stimulates the activity of dermal fibroblasts, the cells deep below the surface that produce collagen. The collagen and elastin fibers continue to multiply after the treatment, and people continue to see improved results over a period of several months.

Nonablative treatments target primarily the skin's color and texture, but early-stage wrinkles may also respond well to nonablative laser treatment. Some nonablative treatments, such as the N-lite laser, target wrinkles more directly. There is preliminary evidence that the N-lite laser may produce a 35 to 55 percent visible improvement of wrinkles after just one treatment.

Lunchtime laser procedures take between fifteen and thirty

Spotlight on Research

REDUCING WRINKLES FROM THE INSIDE OUT

We have had the opportunity to perform a number of studies in our office on the effects of nonablative laser treatments. In one study, appearing in the September 1999 issue of the *Journal of Cutaneous Laser Therapy*, for example, we evaluated the effects of the CoolTouch laser on new collagen formation. Ten subjects with skin types I and II received four treatments each with the CoolTouch laser.

After six months, all ten study participants showed evidence of new dermal collagen formation, and eight reported subjective improvements in the quality of their skin. Such results are significant, because they confirm that it is possible to stimulate new collagen formation without removing the epidermal layers of the skin, as more aggressive facial resurfacing treatments do. Collagen remodeling is essential for reducing facial wrinkles from the inside out.

minutes, and they usually have no side effects. The treatment can be performed on any facial area—around the eyes, mouth, cheeks, chin—with minimal discomfort. A topical anesthetic cream can be used on extra-sensitive areas, but no injections are needed. It is a painless procedure; at most it feels like a rubber band snapping on the skin. After a session, the treated area may appear red for up to an hour; however, makeup can be applied immediately. Since no wound is created, no healing time is required. No one will ever know you have undergone the procedure, people will just tell you how much younger you look and probably ask you what exercise program you're following.

As in the case of Carey, lunchtime laser treatments are becoming popular among people who display fine lines or other early

Nonablative Laser Resurfacing at a Glance

What Does It Do? Improves the quality, tone, and texture of the skin and uneven pigmentation associated with photo damage. Early-stage wrinkles often respond to a nonablative laser treatment. In addition, the treatment is useful as a maintenance procedure following deeper laser resurfacing treatments (see chapter 10).

Skin Types. Nonablative laser resurfacing appears to be safe for all skin types.

Duration of Treatment. About twenty minutes.

Downtime. None; some light redness may occur after the treatment, but it typically disappears after three hours. The only anesthesia used, if needed, is topical.

Risks. In general, nonablative laser treatments are quite safe. Very rarely, scarring may occur.

Number of Treatments Needed. For most lunchtime lasers, up to six treatments spaced about three to four weeks apart is typical. The older the person, the less responsive the skin, so more treatments are required.

How Long Do Results Last? The results presumably last forever. However, because the aging process continues, maintenance treatments at six-month intervals are recommended.

Cost. $500–$1,000/treatment, depending on size of area treated.

signs of photoaging and who want the anti-aging stimulation of new collagen growth induced by the laser light. Generally up to six treatments are needed to generate optimal results. Following this, regular touch-ups are recommended to sustain the growth of new collagen. Because it takes a while for the new collagen growth to become visible on the surface of the skin, the first results will become fully apparent anywhere from three to six months after the procedure.

Nonablative laser treatments appear to be suitable for all skin types. The pigment irregularities induced by traditional laser resurfacing, dermabrasion, or chemical peels generally do not occur with this type of treatment.

Neutralizing Sun Damage with Intense Pulsed Light

Intense Pulsed Light (IPL) technology is another exciting recent arrival on the anti-aging scene. Like the new generation of "lunchtime lasers," Intense Pulsed Light is safe and noninvasive. IPL treatments can erase sun damage and improve the texture of your face and your complexion without disrupting the skin surface. Like nonablative laser treatments, IPL treatments do not entail prolonged recovery time, pain, or potential significant side effects. IPL treatments are sometimes referred to by other names, such as FotoFacial™, EpiFacial™, FacialLight™, and so on.

The hallmark of IPL therapy is its versatility. While laser light emits only one color, or wavelength, at a time, Intense Pulsed Light devices emit many different colors of light. As a result, where most conventional treatment options can address only one problem at a time, IPL can treat several aging issues in the same session. It is the only treatment that can simultaneously address pigmented brown spots, sun damage, enlarged pores, broken capillaries, and other types of skin redness. In addition, IPL treatments stimulate collagen renewal.

Each color of light emitted by IPL machines treats a different problem. Some of the colors remove age spots, others remove flushing and redness of the skin, still others penetrate a bit deeper into the skin and promote new collagen. IPL technology provides an excellent weapon against the cumulative damage wrought by sun exposure and photoaging. It rejuvenates the skin from the inside out by delivering beneficial thermal energy to the deeper layers of the skin.

Whereas the CoolTouch laser, for example, operates in the 1320 nanometer (nm) wavelength, Intense Pulsed Light devices can deliver light in wavelengths ranging from 500 to 1200 nm. The delivered wavelengths can be customized to treat specific problems. Different filters can be used to block certain wavelengths, allowing only light of the desired frequency to reach the target. In general, shorter wavelengths are used to treat skin discoloration, while longer wavelengths actually rejuvenate the skin. In addition, the number and duration of light pulses and the length of the delay between pulses can be customized to deliver the greatest possible effect for each person. This allows the skilled physician to treat several different problems at the same time, while maximizing results and minimizing side effects.

Customizing IPL treatment to the needs of each individual patient is no simple task, and the physician's skill plays a great role in the success of these treatments. Less-experienced professionals sometimes use simpler pulsed light machines that offer fewer choices. The trade-off for greater ease of operation can be less effective treatments and more side effects. In the hands of an experienced practitioner, however, IPL therapy offers a broader range of possibilities than lasers and produces better and more effective results. Examples of powerful IPL machines with a wide range of settings include Photoderm®, Multilight™, EpiLight™, ProLite™, and EsteLux™.

During an IPL treatment, a cold gel is typically applied to the area to be treated. You may be given dark glasses to protect your eyes. The IPL handpiece has a smooth glass surface, which is held to your skin while pulses of light are applied. The most you will

Spotlight on Research

IPL AND WRINKLE REMOVAL

Intense Pulsed Light appears to be highly effective in improving the quality and texture of the skin and creating a more even skin tone. Early research, however, suggests that it may not have as strong an impact on fine lines and wrinkles as other nonablative treatments, such as lasers. While studies done in our office confirm that Intense Pulsed Light does stimulate the formation of new collagen, this may not be sufficient to erase wrinkles. In a study of thirty subjects with mild to moderate wrinkles, twenty-five showed some improvement in the quality of the skin; but even though fine lines and wrinkles were reduced, they did not disappear in any of the subjects.

feel is a slight sting. Few people are bothered by this, but if you find it to be uncomfortable, you can ask the attending physician to apply an anesthetic cream. The treatment is pleasantly relaxing and takes about twenty minutes. A typical treatment program consists of a series of three to six individual treatments — in this way, gradual improvement can be produced with very low risk.

Microdermabrasion

Unlike dermabrasion, its older and more aggressive cousin, microdermabrasion is a gentle, nonablative treatment that removes the outer layer of the skin with a sandblasting technique using aluminum oxide or sodium bicarbonate crystals. The controlled peeling and rapid healing that follow promote renewal of skin

Intense Pulsed Light Treatments at a Glance

What Does It Do? IPL treatments are indicated for individuals who suffer from early signs of photoaging, such as broken capillaries, fine lines and wrinkles, enlarged pores, and mottled pigmentation, including brown spots and freckles. IPL also enhances skin texture and complexion and produces smoother, more youthful skin. It is one of the few anti-aging treatments that can also be used to treat the neck, arms, hands, chest, back, etc. It is also useful for treating rosacea.

Skin Types. IPL appears to be suitable for all skin types.

Duration of Treatment. About twenty minutes.

Downtime. None.

Risks. As with all cosmetic treatments, there is always a slight risk of scarring.

Number of Treatments Needed. The number of treatments needed varies, depending on the number of problems treated, the person's age, and the severity of each condition. A series of three to six treatments is often necessary to produce complete results, and treatments are typically spaced three to four weeks apart.

How Long Do Results Last? Pulsed Light technology is relatively new, but early indications are that results may last for several years.

Cost. $400–$1,500, depending on size of area treated.

surface cells and stimulate the production of new collagen and elastin within the deeper portions of the skin.

Microdermabrasion is becoming increasingly popular. According to the American Society of Plastic Surgeons (ASPS), just over 1 million procedures were performed in the United

Microdermabrasion at a Glance

What Does It Do? Softens fine lines, improves dull and uneven skin color, mitigates clogged pores and blackheads, and promotes production of fresher, more youthful-looking skin. The treatment can also be used on the chest, hands, back, and for rough skin on elbows, knees, and heels.

Skin Types. Suitable for all skin types.

Duration of Treatment. About twenty to forty-five minutes, depending on how large an area is being treated.

Downtime. Your skin may be slightly taut or red immediately after treatment, but you will be able to return to your daily routine without any downtime.

Risks. When done by a medical professional, microdermabrasion is a safe and noninvasive treatment. The treatment is not recommended for people with an acute inflammatory skin condition or for people taking certain medications. In rare cases, some people develop streaking of the skin from the increased blood flow caused by the treatment, but this generally disappears in a day or two.

Number of Treatments Needed. The effects of microdermabrasion treatments are cumulative, and five or more treatment sessions are usually required for optimal results. Treatments are typically performed at intervals of seven to fourteen days.

How Long Do Results Last? Maintenance treatments are required.

Cost. About $150–$250 per treatment, with regional variations.

States in 2001. This treatment helps to erase superficial skin irregularities, especially on the upper lip and crow's-feet areas at the outside corners of the eyes. Treatment of the cheeks and forehead often improves skin color. Microdermabrasion is also useful for acne scars and enlarged pores. The treatment is not usually effective for deep wrinkles, prominent smile lines, or lines that develop from motion, such as frown lines.

Microdermabrasion is often used to complement other skin rejuvenation procedures, such as nonablative lasers or IPL therapy. Because it makes the surface of the skin more absorbent, it can also be used to enhance the effects of therapeutic skin care products.

Before the procedure, your skin is treated with a light cleanser to remove makeup and superficial dust particles. You may be offered goggles to protect your eyes. During the treatment, a small handpiece bombards the surface of the skin with microscopic crystals, wiping off old dead skin cells and leaving a smoother, revitalized skin surface. Afterward, your skin is cleansed again to remove any remaining crystals or dead skin cells. The procedure is usually painless, and there is no need for anesthesia. In addition, there is usually little, if any, immediate evidence that the procedure has been performed, so it imposes no restrictions on work or social activities.

Combined with a comprehensive skin care program that includes age-defying cosmeceuticals, such as AHAs or a tretinoin-based cream, nonablative treatments are important tools to ensure that you enjoy smooth, radiant skin until your late forties and even into your fifties. However, these treatments alone are not enough to ward off the ravages of aging in the second half of your life. Sooner or later it's time to call out the cavalry and pursue more aggressive solutions to combating wrinkles. As the following chapter illustrates, in this area as well, the trend is toward less-invasive treatments that help banish wrinkles from your face with a minimum of discomfort and downtime.

CHAPTER 10

Waging War on Wrinkles

"**B**ut in this world nothing can be said to be certain, except death and taxes," wrote Benjamin Franklin in 1789. Had Franklin lived today, he surely would have added wrinkles to those two unwelcome items on his list. After all, nobody wants them, but everyone gets them. In a culture that worships youth, whatever a wrinkled face may indicate about experience and accumulated wisdom, it is not generally considered attractive. It is no wonder that the battle to dispel the dreaded lines, folds, furrows, and creases takes center stage in the fight against aging. Like it or not, wrinkles date you, and many people consider lines and furrows a liability—socially and professionally.

This was clearly the case for Suzanne. A professional and mother of two in her early forties, Suzanne was showing advanced signs of photoaging when she arrived for her first consultation. The lines around her eyes and mouth had found their groove, so to speak, and had long since set up permanent residence. Her skin was slightly leathery with uneven pigmentation —the result of a penchant for sun worshipping in her younger years. Worries and life experiences she would probably rather have done without had left their mark on her forehead, which was littered with lines that turned into deep furrows whenever she lifted her eyebrows.

Like many professionals, Suzanne was afraid that her aging face was a disadvantage in her job. It didn't help that her company had recently been going through a series of layoffs. Although Suzanne had been spared the ax so far, she was nervous about the possibility of having to compete in the job market with twenty-five-year-year-olds in a not too distant future. In short, Suzanne was ready for a change. When we described how she could improve her appearance with a traditional "laser peel," a deep facial resurfacing treatment, she quickly made up her mind to give it a try.

Because of Suzanne's more advanced stage of aging and sun damage, more powerful skin renewal treatments were necessary. In such cases, lasers that work more deeply are often the treatment of choice. But, as this chapter describes, other treatments, such as chemical peels, dermabrasion, Botox®, and soft-tissue fillers, also afford benefits.

Ablative Laser Resurfacing: CO_2 and Er:YAG

Laser resurfacing is often referred to as a "laser peel" because it uses laser light to vaporize and remove the upper layers of sun-damaged and wrinkled skin. Such deeper-working laser treatment is referred to as *ablative* laser resurfacing. It actually abrades, or scours off, the surface layers of the skin.

A simple principle is at work in all facial resurfacing treatments—the deeper the layers of old, damaged skin peeled off, the greater the potential results in the form of new growth of smoother and more youthful-looking skin. Unfortunately, the deeper the layers of skin that are removed, the deeper is the injury and, hence, the longer and more painful the healing process. While ablative laser treatments are the treatment of choice for deeper wrinkles and advanced photo damage, they are fairly aggressive and involve considerable downtime. In Suzanne's case, she had to schedule her treatment when she could take two vacation weeks to recover from the procedure.

Laser resurfacing, in short, falls into the no-pain, no-gain category of facial rejuvenation therapies. Nonetheless, laser technology presents numerous advantages over more traditional resurfacing treatments, such as deeper chemical peels and dermabrasion. The level of penetration can be controlled more precisely with lasers, so they generally produce less bleeding and postoperative discomfort.

The possibility that lasers could reduce wrinkles was discovered largely by accident. Surgeons noticed that after using lasers to treat acne scars, the skin around the region looked fresher, and wrinkles were less prominent. From such small observations came big possibilities. One of the most important developments in cosmetic laser resurfacing was the introduction of the carbon dioxide (CO_2) laser in the 1990s. The CO_2 laser offered a level of precision, control, and safety that had not been possible with older forms of treatment such as dermabrasion and chemical peels. It soon became the standard laser for use in skin resurfacing, and proved especially useful for people with deep lines or wrinkles, acne scars, or sun-damaged skin. This laser emits a colorless infrared light that targets the water in the skin to remove damaged tissue. The CO_2 laser can cut like a scalpel (it is sometimes referred to as the "surgical laser") but with minimal blood loss. Or it can simply vaporize or ablate tissue, that is, remove the outer layer of skin.

In 1996, there was yet another breakthrough when the Er:YAG laser was introduced. The wavelength of light used in the

Er:YAG laser is readily absorbed by the water in the skin, including water in damaged collagen. The laser light heats the water, creating a mild thermal injury. As this injury heals, new, thicker, and more regular collagen replaces the old photo-damaged collagen fibers. The Er:YAG laser generally does not penetrate as deeply into the skin as the CO_2 laser does. As a result, it provides a gentler treatment than the CO_2 laser with less associated thermal damage. With the Er:YAG laser, there is less risk of scarring and burns, less pain, and faster recovery time. The Er:YAG laser has proved to be the best choice for people without very deep lines, with moderate acne scars and age spots, and for those who want to improve the overall texture of their skin.

The CO_2 and Er:YAG lasers are often used in combination, according to what is best for each skin problem treated. This is what we did in Suzanne's case. The CO_2 laser wavelength was used to treat the deep wrinkles around her mouth by removing the outer layers of sun-damaged, aging skin, while the wavelengths emitted by the Er:YAG were used for the thinner skin around her eyes.

During a laser treatment, the laser is moved back and forth over the skin until the desired level of exposure has been reached. More localized treatments focusing just on wrinkles around the mouth or eyes can be done without sedation, using a topical anesthetic cream and perhaps a small amount of local anesthesia. However, a treatment like Suzanne's, which involved the whole face, requires general anesthesia. The procedure is done on an outpatient basis, but you need to have someone drive you home after the treatment.

Like most people, Suzanne had to use painkillers after the procedure to reduce postoperative discomfort. Although she was initially dismayed by the swelling, oozing, redness, and peeling she experienced, she realized that it was a normal part of the healing process. We gave her several protective ointments to facilitate healing and recovery.

Suzanne's face healed without complications, and after two weeks she returned to work. It took a while for the remaining redness of her skin to subside, but she told her colleagues that she had gotten a bad sunburn on her vacation. When she came for a follow-up visit a few months later, she was thrilled with the dramatic decrease in the wrinkles around her eyes and mouth and the smooth, pinkish, youthful skin that was gradually replacing the leathery, unevenly textured skin we had removed. All the discomfort of the first two weeks following the procedure had been forgotten.

The results of laser resurfacing are not permanent, but they last considerably longer than less invasive, nonablative procedures. In Suzanne's case, we prescribed a topical tretinoin cream to contribute to her continued improvement. We also used Botox injections (described in greater detail in chapter 11) to further smooth out the furrows in her forehead. In addition, we recommended that she have regular nonablative procedures as a follow-up to prolong the effects of the laser peel.

Electrosurgical Resurfacing: Coblation

Coblation, a promising new technique for facial resurfacing, offers many of the benefits of deep laser resurfacing with the potential for reduced discomfort and quicker healing time. Although approved only recently as a skin treatment in the United States, coblation has been used for facial resurfacing in Australia for several years.

Originally developed to resurface joint cartilage, coblation uses kinetic energy to disrupt the molecular bonds of the skin cells and remove damaged skin tissue. Where lasers apply the heat energy generated by light waves to resurface the skin, coblation — or "cold ablation" — uses a microelectrical radio frequency. This technology affords safer and gentler treatment for two reasons. First, because

Ablative Laser Resurfacing at a Glance

What Does It Do? Laser resurfacing with the CO_2 or Er:YAG lasers is the treatment of choice for the deeper wrinkles and uneven pigmentation associated with advanced sun damage.

Skin Type. The treatment works best on fair skin.

Duration of Treatment. Anywhere from a few minutes to ninety minutes, depending on how large an area is treated.

Downtime. Most people need one to two weeks off to recover enough to return to their normal routine. The crusts formed on the skin in the treated area usually peel off after ten days, and it may take up to six months for the skin redness to subside. Initially the skin will be much more sensitive to sunlight after the procedure, so careful precautions must be taken to protect your skin from the sun.

Risks. In the hands of an inexperienced practitioner, the laser may give off too much heat, causing burns or scarring. Lasers can also create uneven pigmentation, that is, a lightening or darkening of the treated skin. In rare cases, laser resurfacing may activate herpes virus infections (cold sores).

Number of Treatments Needed. One treatment usually suffices. If wrinkles are very deep or sun damage severe, your physician may recommend that treatment be spread out over more than one session.

How Long Do Results Last? It takes several months for the full results of laser resurfacing to appear. Once the redness fades, people typically report a significant improvement in their appearance, which lasts for several years as long as proper sun protection is maintained. However, natural movements of the face eventually cause expression lines to recur.

Cost. The average national cost is $3,500–$8,000

Coblation at a Glance

What Does It Do? Coblation is used primarily for wrinkles and other signs of photodamage, such as mottled pigmentation. It is most suitable for patients in their mid-twenties to mid-forties, who have mild to moderate skin damage and wrinkles. Since it removes the epidermal layer of the skin, it is also useful for treating age spots and precancerous cell growth. Coblation shows promise in the treatment of scars as well.

Skin Types. Preliminary results indicate that coblation is safe for use on most skin types.

Duration of Treatment. Between fifteen and sixty minutes.

Downtime. Usually four to eight days.

Risks. The risk of scarring seen with all cosmetic procedures.

Number of Treatments Needed. Usually one.

How Long Do Results Last? Generally more than one year.

Cost. $500–$2,000, depending on the size of the area being treated.

radio frequencies, and not heat energy, are used to peel away facial tissue, there is generally less thermal tissue damage to surrounding areas. Second, coblation affords more precise control, disintegrating skin tissue layer by layer and minimizing unwanted damage. As a consequence, when performed correctly, this treatment can be very safe and provide more predictable results. Unlike laser treatments and dermabrasion, bleeding rarely occurs.

The recovery period after a coblation treatment is usually dramatically shorter than after laser resurfacing. Like all resurfacing procedures, however, the treatment creates redness, and mild to moderate swelling may also develop. However, the swelling generally subsides within a week, at which time makeup can be

Special Considerations for Ethnic Skin

Until recently, people of ethnic background had few options for ablative resurfacing treatments, such as laser resurfacing, dermabrasion, and chemical peels. The darker skin of people with skin types V–VI is more likely to develop abnormal pigmentation as a result of the injury caused when the outer layers of skin are removed. To some extent, this drawback is made up for by the fact that people with darker skin are less susceptible to UV damage. However, photoaging does occur in dark skin, most commonly showing up as pigmentation irregularities, freckles, or redness.

People with darker skin may develop several problems in response to traditional resurfacing treatments. One of the most common is *hypopigmentation,* in which there is a loss of skin color in the treated area. Another common response is *hyperpigmentation,* or increased skin color. People of African or Mediterranean ancestry are also more likely to develop *keloidal scars,* "ropy," raised scars that occur as an abnormal healing response to skin injury.

Nonablative resurfacing procedures, such as lunchtime laser treatments, typically produce excellent results in ethnic skin. Until recently, however, deeper laser resurfacing treatments were not generally recommended. Fortunately, a number of treatments have emerged

(continued on next page)

applied. Unlike laser resurfacing, where redness may linger for up to six months, residual redness usually disappears in less time.

Coblation does not replace laser resurfacing; rather, it presents an alternative that falls somewhere between nonablative and ablative resurfacing techniques. The results are not as deep and compre-

Special Considerations for Ethnic Skin (continued)

in recent years that appear to address the specific needs of ethnic skin with far less risk. Coblation techniques using radio frequency waves instead of heat waves appear to be relatively safer for ethnic skin. In addition, there is evidence that the less aggressive Er:YAG laser may be safe for Asian skin. In a 1998 study, we evaluated fifty individuals of Asian heritage. We found that the Er:YAG laser could be used safely to treat wrinkles, scars, and pigment changes.

Finally, a recently introduced modified version of the CO_2 laser, known as the UltraPulse® Encore™ System with CO_2 Lite™, has helped to expand the possibilities available for ethnic skin. The UltraPulse Encore system gives greater depth control, and the CO_2 Lite feature provides greater control over the amount of heat delivered to the tissue during treatment, thereby reducing the risk of adverse results in ethnic skin.

Lasers are also used with great success to treat skin conditions prevalent in ethnic populations. Many African- or Asian-Americans, for example, develop small, hyperpigmented bumps on the face, a condition known as *dermatosis papulosa nigra*. These bumps can be removed successfully with a variable-pulsed KTP laser. Similarly, the bluish-colored skin lesions common in Asians, known as *nevus of Ota*, can be treated with lasers.

hensive as those of ablative techniques, but they are considerably greater than for nonablative procedures. The long-term effects of coblation have yet to be demonstrated, but so far it appears to have positive results. We recently studied the microscopic changes induced by coblation and found that treatment led to the formation of new, young, and immature collagen, which eventually was transformed into healthy, mature collagen. This study explains why people's skin looks younger after coblation treatments.

A Nonsurgical Facelift

Another promising new treatment using radio frequency instead of laser light is ThermaCool TC™ (or Thermalift). ThermaCool TC shows promise as a noninvasive means of achieving some of the same results that would be gained through the surgery associated with traditional facelifts.

While facial resurfacing treatments improve the quality, tone, and texture of the skin, none provides the skin tightening seen with a facelift or browlift. During the ThermaCool procedure, radio frequencies are applied to the deeper layers of skin tissue to produce a tightening of the skin in certain areas. By tightening the skin on the forehead, for example, eyebrows are raised slightly, which makes the eyes look less droopy and more open and alert. Similarly, sagging skin on the cheeks and neck can be tightened, reducing the deep folds that appear as you get older.

The treatment lasts for five to twenty minutes, depending on how large an area is being treated. The most you feel is a brief sensation of heat each time the machine is fired. Typically, an anesthetic cream is applied before the procedure to minimize discomfort.

There is usually no downtime after the treatment, and the most common side effect is a slight redness, which vanishes within an hour or two. Based on preliminary results, adverse effects are rare with this type of treatment.

Results develop as the tissue in the deeper layers of the skin gradually regenerates, so it takes at least a month for effects to emerge and four to six months before full results are visible.

Although never expected to provide the same results as a facelift, this exciting new technology does provide a skin-tightening alternative to those who wish to avoid extensive surgery. The procedure is generally performed with topical anesthetic cream and causes no wounding. It too can be done during a lunchtime break!

The Downside of Laser Technology

In the hands of a qualified practitioner, laser treatments are among the safest skin treatments available today. However, lasers are powerful tools and must be used carefully and with skill. While nonablative lasers are relatively risk-free and easy to work with, more powerful lasers, particularly the CO_2 laser systems, are more difficult to master. This can be a significant problem, because inappropriately administered laser treatments can lead to severe burns and long-term scarring.

If you are opting for any laser procedure, especially laser resurfacing, you must take great care in selecting a practitioner. There is no nationally regulated credentialing for people planning to practice laser surgery, and state regulations vary widely. As a result, many inexperienced or unqualified practitioners have entered the field over the last few years. Some laser manufacturers provide one- or two-day training courses for would-be practitioners. In a number of states, family doctors, obstetricians, and even dentists and massage therapists with a minimum of training and experience now offer laser surgery. Treatment is often also available at spas and "wellness centers." The onus, therefore, is on patients to educate themselves about the qualifications of the practitioner.

Most of the medical laser market in the United States is rental. Many physicians renting such lasers do only a few laser procedures

Thermalift at a Glance

What Does It Do? Lifts sagging skin by tightening the skin on the forehead, cheeks, or neck. It is most suitable for patients in their mid-thirties to mid-fifties with moderate skin sagging.

Skin Types. Preliminary results indicate that the treatment is safe for use on most skin types.

Duration of Treatment. About five to twenty minutes.

Downtime. None.

Risks. Initial results indicate that the treatment is unusually safe. Long-term effects are not known.

Number of Treatments Needed. Generally two to four.

How Long Do Results Last? One or two "touch-up" treatments are typically recommended every twelve to eighteen months.

Cost. $1,000–$2,000 per treatment.

each month. That is not necessarily good news for patients. Although it is unfair to generalize, many rental laser machines are transported by vans that bounce around and can damage the equipment. Many such machines also tend to be older and not well tuned. Someone using a rental laser may not know how old it is or when its last tune-up was. Think of the difference between a rental car and a car you own. Which one has been cared for so that it functions safely and effectively? The contrast between purchased lasers used at full-time laser centers and daily laser rental units used by the occasional laser physician should be obvious.

If a laser practitioner rents a machine, the implication is that he or she is not engaged in full-time or even frequent laser surgery. The physician also may not be well versed in the correct procedures. That can spell real problems. Being a once-in-a-while laser surgeon is like trying to be an electrician on the weekends after having taken a few short courses sometime in the past. Each laser is unique and requires specialized knowledge and hours of hands-on experience. Up to thirty lasers may be used, and they are all different. As with any surgical procedure, there is no room for error. Lasers are potent tools, and in the hands of the novice user, they can wreak serious damage to the skin and cause severe burns and scarring.

The good news, however, is that although the risks are real, they can be controlled by taking systematic steps to find a qualified physician. Don't just go to the *Yellow Pages* and pick out whoever has the nicest-looking advertisement. You should not be shy about inquiring about the practitioner's qualifications and experience. Ask direct questions and listen to the answers. After all, it's your skin that's going to be affected by the procedure. You need to have confidence in the person you are selecting to treat you. If you have doubts, find someone else.

Other Resurfacing Procedures: Dermabrasion and Chemical Peels

DERMABRASION

This treatment was developed originally in 1905, but poor results caused it to be abandoned until 1953. That year, new technology emerged that provided better control and safety. Dermabrasion was one of the first treatments developed to correct many of the signs of sun damage and aging and improve the appearance of certain types of scars.

The standard dermabrasion technique employs a small hand-held electrically powered device that rotates a wire brush or

The Informed Consumer

HOW TO CHOOSE AN EXPERIENCED AND QUALIFIED LASER PRACTITIONER

The first rule of thumb is to use only a board-certified dermatologist or other appropriately trained laser surgeon. Certification by the American Board of Dermatology means that the doctor has undergone extensive training and a rigorous examination in dermatology, including medical school, internship, and at least a three-year dermatology residency. You need to be careful because, in most states, a doctor is permitted to call himself or herself a dermatologist without being board-certified.

The second rule is, be informed and ask lots of questions. You must find out about the doctor's credentials. Questions you should ask include:

- What kind of training have you had?
- Where did you study and receive certification?
- How long have you been performing this procedure and on how many patients?
- What were the results?
- Did they incur any short- or long-term problems?
- How many different kinds of treatment have you performed?
- Do you own or rent your laser equipment?
- How many lasers do you use? Two or three, or twenty to twenty-five?
- Have you published or lectured on lasers?

Always ask for professional referrals, names of satisfied patients, and before-and-after photos. You should feel comfortable with the doctor you choose—and you should both have the same expectations. As long as you do your homework and make an informed choice of surgeon, you have every chance of getting the results you desire. Find out about qualified laser physicians from the American Society for Laser Medicine and Surgery or the American Society for Dermatologic Surgery.

Dermabrasion at a Glance

What Does It Do? Dermabrasion has traditionally been used for treating deep wrinkles.

Skin Types. Because dermabrasion may permanently lighten or discolor the skin, it is not recommended for African-Americans or American-Asians or anyone with dark skin.

Duration of Treatment. Depending on how much skin is to be treated, the procedure may take anywhere from a few minutes to an hour and a half.

Downtime. For a full face treatment, temporary swelling, itching, or redness occurs. Most people are able to return to work after two weeks.

Risks. Scarring and pigmentary changes of the face.

Number of Treatments Needed. Usually one treatment suffices; in severe cases, more than one session may be required.

How Long Do Results Last? The treatment permanently removes existing wrinkles, but does not prevent new ones from forming over time.

Cost. $1,500–$4,000 depending on size of area treated.

diamond-coated stainless steel wheel at speeds of 15,000–30,000 rpm. It scrapes away the outer layer of the skin and makes wrinkles disappear or at least less noticeable. By using a combination of oral sedatives, local anesthetics, injections of narcotic pain medications, and topical spray refrigerants, the procedure can be done in an outpatient setting. It can also be used in conjunction with other procedures, such as chemical peels.

Dermabrasion of the full face involves considerable downtime. Temporary swelling, itching, or redness occurs, but most people are able to return to work after two weeks and resume full activities in four to six weeks. Redness may persist for up to three months, and you will need to wait six months to a year before going out in the sun for any length of time, even with appropriate sunscreen.

CHEMICAL PEELS

This type of treatment uses a variety of chemical agents to peel off the top layer of skin and improve wrinkles. There are light (also called superficial), medium, and deep peel treatments.

A light peel is relatively harmless and is often performed by an esthetician. Most light peels use alpha hydroxy acid (AHA) preparations with a considerably stronger concentration than that found in over-the-counter cosmetic products. A light peel does a great job at temporarily smoothing rough, dry skin and fine wrinkles. It requires no anesthetic, and the only discomfort is a mild stinging sensation. After the peel, you may experience mild flaking, scaling, redness, and dry skin, but this does not last long or prevent you from resuming your regular activities. Several treatments may be necessary to create significant results, but you can maintain the results by using an over-the-counter AHA product, mixed with a skin cream.

If you are getting a light peel through an esthetician, be sure he or she is licensed. AHA peels used by estheticians often have concentrations of 20 to 35 percent, and the person applying the peel needs to have proper training in application and sanitation procedures. Some dermatologists and cosmetic surgeons regard AHA peels as unsafe in the hands of practitioners without any medical training. Although light peels are relatively innocuous, you want to avoid them if you have facial warts, cold sores, or are pregnant or lactating. The same applies if you are taking Accutane®, have a sunburn or allergies to the sun, or have recently had facial surgery.

Chemical Peels at a Glance

What Does It Do? A chemical peel removes the surface layers of the skin, creating a smoother, fresher-looking skin surface and erasing wrinkles. The deeper the peel, the more extensive the skin renewal. Medium and deep peels stimulate collagen renewal, resulting in firmer skin and diminished wrinkles.

Skin Types. Both light and medium peels are considered safe for people with dark skin. African-American skin has a greater buildup of dead skin cells, which can create a dull look and clog pores. Light peels are very effective at counteracting this problem. Deep peels are not suitable for ethnic skin types.

Duration of Treatment. Light and medium peels take from thirty to sixty minutes, and are performed without anesthesia. A deep peel often takes two hours, and a painkiller or light sedation is needed.

Downtime. There is little or no downtime for light peels. For a medium-depth peel, you'll need to take at least four to seven days off work, while a deep peel entails at least two weeks of downtime.

Risks. Both medium and deep peels carry risk of scarring because the chemicals can burn the skin if they are left on for too long. This risk is most significant for a deep peel. Deep peels cause a permanent change in skin color; the face takes on an irreversible pallor. Postoperative infections can cause unexpected complications.

Number of Treatments Needed. A light peel typically requires repeated applications. For a medium or deep peel, one treatment usually suffices.

How Long Do Results Last? In general, the deeper the peel, the longer the effect. A light peel must be repeated regularly, while a medium peel will last up to a year. A deep peel will create permanent results, although new wrinkles may form.

Cost. A light peel costs $75 and up; a medium peel is $1,000 and up; and a deep peel is $2,000–$4,000, depending on the size of the area treated.

A medium peel creates more extensive skin renewal and stimulates collagen to firm the skin and improve wrinkles in the months following the peel. This type of peel is performed with a stronger chemical agent, which removes a thicker layer of skin. Common agents used in this type of peel are trichloroacetic acid (TCA) in 20–50 percent strength and Jessner's solution, which is a mixture of acids. A medium peel smoothes crow's-feet and mild to moderate wrinkles and corrects superficial blemishes and pigmentation problems. It may also remove precancerous lesions. You may experience tingling or throbbing that can be relieved with a painkiller, and there may also be swelling, but it subsides within a week. There is a small risk of scarring.

For a deep peel, the solution used is generally phenol (carbolic acid), a coal tar derivative. It is the most effective form of peel, penetrating deeply into the skin. It can remove deeper wrinkles and treat other advanced signs of sun damage. A deep peel is serious business, so you should educate yourself well before choosing this extremely aggressive treatment. The procedure can take two hours to perform, and the patient is usually given painkillers and sedated. Some people may need a one- or two-day hospital stay, and a two-week absence from work is common. Potential serious medical problems may arise from deep chemical peels. For the first few days, the face may be swollen, and the eyes may even be swollen shut. A liquid diet may be needed for several days, and talking is difficult. Within seven to ten days, new red skin will form, but it takes weeks before it attains normal skin color. You should be able to return to normal activities about two weeks after treatment, at which time you can apply makeup.

The good news about a deep peel is that only one treatment is necessary to achieve results, and those results are permanent. New wrinkles will develop over time, of course, and the treated skin will be lighter than before and usually will not tan. A deep peel leaves the skin extremely sensitive to the sun, so proper sun protection is crucial.

CHAPTER 11

Fashioning the Face of the Future

*A*nyone living in America today can hardly have failed to notice the media attention given to the botulinum toxin type A, or Botox, as it is popularly called. Arriving on the anti-aging scene only five years ago, Botox has quickly become extremely popular. In 2001, more than 1.6 million Botox procedures were performed on about 850,000 patients. The number of people receiving Botox injections is expected to quadruple over the next five years.

While facial resurfacing treatments remove old, damaged skin to stimulate the growth of new, younger-looking skin, Botox is part of a family of antiwrinkle treatments that use an entirely different strategy. These remedies use an external agent to fill out folds and creases or to relax muscles that create wrinkles and expression lines.

The advantage of these wrinkle treatments is that they can produce radical results, yet they are about as fast, painless, and convenient as having your hair done. They also involve little risk when performed correctly and little or no healing process or downtime. The disadvantage of these treatments is that the effects in most cases are relatively short-lived, and they need to be repeated regularly. The body's natural processes break down foreign elements over time, making the effects of the treatment disappear after as little as three to four months.

Smoothing Wrinkles with Botox

Botox is a neurotoxin derived from the bacterium causing botulism, a type of food poisoning that can develop in improperly sealed cans or other stored foods. While botulism can be extremely dangerous, causing generalized paralysis and even death if not treated in time, the purified version of the botulism toxin used in Botox is so diluted that it is completely harmless. The Federal Drug Administration recently approved Botox for the treatment of frown lines, but doctors also use it to treat forehead lines, crow's-feet, and a variety of other wrinkles. Long before it became a cosmetic wonder child, Botox was used to treat a number of eye conditions, including eye-muscle twitching, excessive blinking, and cross-eye. It is also prescribed for severe head and neck pain, chronic migraine and tension headaches, and excessive sweating. The virtues of the product for wrinkle treatment were discovered only recently, but the procedure affords such an easy way to smooth out wrinkles that it rapidly has become one of the leading wrinkle treatments.

Botox is quick, easy, and fairly painless. To treat wrinkles, a tiny amount of Botox is injected directly into a specific facial muscle, for example, between the brows, causing the muscle that creates the wrinkle to relax. Since the muscle can no longer contract, the wrinkle disappears like magic. With a smooth forehead,

Botox at a Glance

What Does It Do? Botox affords an easy and relatively painless way to erase expression lines caused by contracted muscles, such as crow's-feet, forehead furrows, frown lines, and neck creases.

Duration of Treatment. About five to fifteen minutes, depending on the number of injections.

Downtime. None; you can go back to work immediately. Results take four to seven days to become fully visible.

Risks. When used by a skilled practitioner, Botox has an excellent safety record. In the hands of an unskilled practitioner, excessive injection of Botox can temporarily disable certain facial expressions or cause facial asymmetry.

Number of Treatments Needed. Two to ten injections are typical for the first treatment.

How Long Do Results Last? Results from the first injections last three to four months. After several treatments , injections may last longer, about five to six months.

Cost. $300–$2,000, depending on the number of injections required.

it looks like you have never had a worry or a frown in your life. Yes, results can sometimes be as dramatic as this.

Treatment with Botox takes only a short time and works within about forty-eight to ninety-six hours. The big drawback is that its beneficial effects are short-lived. After about three or four months, the treated facial muscles regain their mobility, and wrinkles start to reappear. In short, regular, ongoing treatments are necessary to retain the anti-aging benefits of Botox.

Beauty Secrets of the Rich and Famous

Ever wondered how daytime soap opera stars manage to remain so young and restless, so bold and beautiful? Many of these shows are well into their second decade, yet their leading stars somehow seem miraculously untouched by Father Time.

Chalk it up to the advances of modern cosmetic dermatology. Soft-tissue fillers, Botox, Gore-Tex® implants, and other treatments that can change the appearance of the face dramatically without painful and expensive surgery have long since joined mascara, foundation, and blush in the beauty arsenal of actors and actresses.

Some female stars opt for treatments that create fuller, more sensuous lips—the so-called Paris Pout, a look created by injections with cow collagen or other fillers. But if anything has caught the fancy of Tinseltown, it is Botox.

"We keep Botox in the refrigerator," says *That's Life* star Heather Paige Kent to a reporter at Hollywood.com. "My husband is a plastic surgeon, and he injects me every six months."

Stars may love the stuff, but according to the *New York Times*, directors like Martin Scorcese and Baz Luhrman grumble that Botox-saturated stars are losing their ability to emote. Oh, well. Who is to say that beauty doesn't come at a cost?

The skill of the person doing the injection plays a considerable role in the results. Anyone with an M.D. can inject the shots, but it takes training and experience to administer the shots properly. If not injected properly, Botox can cause drooping eyelids, sagging mouth, or facial asymmetry. This happens when the injection also affects the neighboring muscles, which become weak. Fortunately, such side effects wear off within a few weeks.

Botox works only for motion or expression wrinkles, such as frowns and crow's-feet. For deep creases, it may not be enough and will have to be supplemented with another treatment, typically a filler agent. Botox does not work for some wrinkles in the lower part of the face that are caused by aging instead of muscle contraction. In addition, it cannot be used for smile lines, since you need these muscles to eat and to form facial expressions.

Some experts are wary of Botox and warn that people who use it will no longer be able to produce the facial expressions that are essential to human communication. For example, think of the number of times frown lines come in handy when you want to let your kids (or anyone else) know that you are not the least bit pleased with them. But the warnings are probably unnecessary. Even fresh from a Botox treatment, you can still raise your eyebrows, which conveys a great deal, and the notion that you can only express your mood or emotion with the help of wrinkles is somewhat questionable.

Myobloc® (botulinum toxin type B), a recently developed alternative to Botox, produces similar effects more quickly—within forty-eight hours, as opposed to the forty-eight to ninety-six hours for Botox injections. However, the effects of Myobloc appear not to last as long; they begin to wear off after eight weeks, rather than the three to four months Botox typically lasts. Doctors are experimenting with different Myobloc dosages, and other botulinum toxins, to try to match the effects of Botox.

Collagen-Based Soft-Tissue Fillers

The principle behind this antiwrinkle treatment is simple—delay or reverse the decline of collagen that results in wrinkles by injecting collagen into the dermis to plump up the skin and smooth out wrinkles. Unlike Botox, collagen injections are effective for wrinkles that are present when the face is in repose—that is, wrinkles that don't derive from facial expressions.

Collagen Injections at a Glance

What Does It Do? Collagen erases furrows and creases by plumping up dermal tissue. Collagen injections are most commonly used for wrinkles and folds on the lower part of the face.

Duration of Treatment. Ten to twenty minutes.

Downtime. None.

Risks. Collagen injected too close to the surface may create a "bumpy" look. If the collagen is injected too deeply, the effect only lasts a few weeks.

Number of Treatments Needed. One initial treatment suffices, but touch-ups are required every three to six months.

How Long Do Results Last? Three to four months.

Costs. Collagen-based filling treatments average $300–$1,000 per session, depending on the type of collagen used and how much filling material is injected.

A number of different types of collagen treatments are available. One of the most common is *bovine collagen,* sold under the brand names Zyplast® and Zyderm®. For this treatment, collagen is derived from cows and purified to make it resemble human collagen. Collagen treatment with animal collagen requires two skin tests beforehand, since some people are allergic to it, and there will be a wait of about four weeks to see if there is any adverse reaction.

Human collagen fillers are often used for people who are allergic to animal collagen. Fillers such as Dermalogen™, Cymetra®, or

Alloderm® use collagen protein or other human tissue harvested from human cadavers. Although not for the squeamish, these fillers are not allergenic, and they are, to some extent, capable of regenerating normal tissue.

Soft-tissue augmentation involves injections at the site of wrinkles; it causes only mild discomfort. Improvement occurs almost immediately after a collagen injection and last up to six months. By then the collagen has been broken down by the body's own enzymes, and the procedure has to be repeated. As the lines in your face deepen with age, collagen gradually loses effectiveness, and you need more frequent injections, as often as every two weeks. At that point, it is time to look to other treatments to address your beauty concerns.

Autologous Fat Transfer

Autologous fat transfer (microlipoinjection) is typically used when a more permanent filler for wrinkles is desired. In this procedure, fat is taken from the patient's own body, usually from the thighs, buttocks, or stomach, and reinjected into the wrinkles below the skin. Because the filler is taken from the patient's own body, there is no chance of allergic reaction. While early results indicated that fat injections in the face were reabsorbed too easily, recently developed techniques for harvesting and injecting fat create longer-lasting effects.

This technique is best suited for reducing deep wrinkles, such as the nasolabial folds around the mouth. This type of filler becomes a particularly attractive alternative as you get older and other fillers get prohibitively expensive, because more and more is needed to create the same results.

Repeated treatments are needed, although research published in the June 2002 *Archives of Dermatology* suggests that an improvement

Fat Injections at a Glance

What Does It Do? Bulkier than collagen, fat is excellent for plumping up the deeper lines generally apparent from the late thirties and onward.

Duration of Treatment. About thirty to sixty minutes.

Downtime. None.

Risks. Fat transfer is generally safe. Unlike collagen injections, no allergic reaction is possible because material from your own body is used.

Number of Treatments Needed. Generally one treatment brings about the desired results.

How Long Do Results Last? The results build up over time, but plan on needing touch-up injections every six months.

Cost. About $1,000–$2,000 for the first treatment, during which fat is removed from the body and injected into the desired area. Extra fat can be stored and used for future injections, which typically run $150–$300 per injection.

lasting more than a year is possible. Generally, each procedure results in 15 to 20 percent permanent improvement with touch-ups needed about every six months.

Gore-Tex

This synthetic substance is threaded under the skin, pushing the wrinkle up. It has been shown to be particularly effective for the nasolabial folds around the mouth area, but it is also used in cheek, lip, and chin augmentation. There may be some swelling after the treatment, but side effects are rare.

Gore-Tex at a Glance

What Does It Do? Augments chin, cheeks, or lips, or permanently removes the nasolabial lines that typically become a problem in the early to late forties.

Duration of Treatment. About thirty to sixty minutes.

Downtime. None.

Risks. Gore-Tex doesn't move with your expressions, so you will be able to feel it under the skin, particularly when you talk. Occasionally, implants may migrate in which case they can be removed only through surgery.

Number of Treatments Needed. One.

How Long Do Results Last? Gore-Tex implants create permanent results.

Cost. $1,500–$2,000.

Gore-Tex stands out among fillers because the results are permanent. But it can only be used to fill lines in the lower third of the face, specifically the nasolabial lines. The material is like a spaghetti strand; it is threaded under the skin and attached to the top and bottom of the nasolabial line.

A New Generation of Soft-Tissue Fillers

The race to develop soft-tissue fillers that create more permanent results has given rise to a slew of new products. Some of these have gained FDA approval for use in the United States, while numerous others are in the approval process.

Mostly for Men

Although the majority of people who undergo cosmetic treatments are women, men are turning to such procedures in increasing numbers. Many men believe that continuing to look youthful and attractive is important for career success. They do not want to be perceived as losing their edge just because they are getting older.

According to the American Society of Plastic Surgeons, 48,400 men had collagen injections in the United States in 2001, up from 39,075 in 1999 and 24,810 in 1997. Botox is catching on among men, too. Of the 850,000 patients receiving Botox treatments last year, an estimated 12 percent, or more than 100,000, were men.

But the most popular treatment by far for men is the chemical peel. In 2001, 168,093 men underwent this procedure, more than double the 1999 figure of 82,221, which was itself almost three times the 1997 figure. Laser treatments were also popular, with 129,722 men undergoing laser hair removal, and laser treatment of facial veins was also a common procedure.

Once they have decided on cosmetic surgical treatment, men tend to experience the process in a very different way from women. According to E. Bingo Wyer, in *The Unofficial Guide to Cosmetic Surgery*, research shows that men require more anesthetic, disregard postoperative requirements, have less patience with the process, and have a lower threshold of pain.

Hmmm. A case of lies, damned lies, and statistics?

Artecoll® is an exciting new collagen-based filler that promises to create more durable results than previous collagen fillers. Artecoll has long been used in Canada to smooth out wrinkles and acne scars and to plump up lips. The filler consists of plastic microspheres suspended in a solution of bovine collagen and 0.3 percent lidocaine (for pain relief). Unlike collagen injections, which work almost immediately, it takes three months for the full effects of Artecoll to manifest. During this time, the injected collagen is absorbed by the body and replaced by new collagen the body creates. The new collagen binds to the microspheric plastic beads, keeping them in place and creating an effect that lasts far longer than traditional collagen injections.

Another new and exciting type of soft-tissue filler in the pipeline is based on hyaluronic acid, the main water-binding agent in the dermal ground substance that helps plump up the skin. Fillers based on hyaluronic acid have been used successfully in Europe and Canada since 1998, and a number of them are in the process of gaining FDA approval. Hyaluronic acid-based products such as DermaLive® and Dermadeep® have been shown to produce long-lasting positive results as much as three years after the treatment. Unlike fillers containing animal ingredients, no allergy test is needed. Among the most popular fillers likely to be available soon are Restylane®, Perlane®, and Hylaform®, also based on hyaluronic acid.

Your Anti-Aging Arsenal through the Decades

Your best bet for retaining a youthful appearance is to start early with a combination of good skin care and anti-aging treatments to combat the milder signs of aging. As you grow older, more treatments should be added to your anti-aging arsenal to deal with more advanced signs of aging. At its website, the American Society for Dermatologic Surgery recommends the following steps.

- **In Your 20s.** In the buoyant twenties, long-term skin care may be the last thing on your mind. Although you're likely to enjoy the most beautiful skin you will ever have, this is typically the age at which cosmetic flaws first appear, such as fine lines and freckles, particularly if you're not getting appropriate sun protection. In addition to a good daily skin care regimen, preventive anti-aging care at this stage includes regular light chemical peels and—particularly in the second half of this decade—nonablative resurfacing techniques, such as "lunchtime lasers," microdermabrasion, and Intense Pulsed Light.

- **In Your 30s.** This is the decade when you are forced to realize that you, too, will grow older one day. Crow's-feet around the eyes, furrows in the forehead, the first signs of lines around the mouth, and brown spots or mottled pigmentation are some of this decade's common aging markers. If the signs of aging are not too dramatic, nonablative resurfacing techniques suffice for this decade as well. You should also consider using a tretinoin-based cream, such as Renova or Retin-A. For more pesky lines and furrows, you may want to try coblation, Botox, light chemical peels, and soft-tissue fillers.

- **In Your 40s.** You're likely to be at the top of your form in this decade, old enough to experience significant career success and family fulfillment and young enough to enjoy it. At this point, wrinkles and folds have likely set up permanent residence around your eyes, forehead, and mouth, and you may have developed baggy eyelids and sagging jowls. Age spots and other pigmentation problems are also typical companions at this age. This is the time to step up the treatments you are already using and consider adding laser resurfacing, pigment-specific brown spot lasers, and medium chemical peels to your anti-aging arsenal.

- **In Your 50s and Beyond.** If you have taken good care of your skin in previous decades, this is the time when you'll really reap the results in the form of smooth, radiant, youthful skin. However, even if you didn't, there are many ways to combat the deep lines and wrinkles, pigmentation changes, and loose skin common at this age. The best results are often achieved by combining a number of different treatments. A skilled cosmetic dermatologist or dermatological surgeon can help you to develop a plan for achieving a safe mix and match of techniques without having to resort to invasive surgery.

CHAPTER 12

Common Beauty Concerns and Their Treatment

When most people fantasize about what they would do with a small windfall, a skiing trip or a vacation to Hawaii is likely to rank right up there along with a new car. Getting laser treatments for a skin problem is not likely to top the list, or even make it there at all. However, there was no doubt in Laura's mind that this was exactly how to earmark part of a small inheritance from her mother.

"I had been suffering from acne for a long time, and I found the scars to be terribly disfiguring," explains Laura. "I would try to cover them with makeup, but it just wasn't enough."

Laura had married recently, and although her husband said he didn't care about the scars, she felt self-conscious about her appearance and wanted to look her best for him. She had read that lasers can improve acne scars, but her budget was tight. Until now. "When this money came along, it just seemed the perfect opportunity," says Laura. "I figured, 'Hey, a windfall is a windfall.'"

As is common among people with severe cases of acne, Laura's face was covered with numerous scars of different sizes and depth, including ice-pick (small and deep) and saucerized (wide and shallow) scars. She preferred a gentle treatment, so we used the Smoothbeam laser to gently erase the scars on her face. The laser stimulates the formation of new collagen in the deeper layers of skin and raises depressed scars by improving the collagen fibers deep in the skin.

It took six treatments over a three-month period to smooth the scars on Laura's cheeks and chin, and another four months before the results became fully visible. As new, rosy, and greatly improved skin gradually replaced some of the potholes on her cheeks, Laura was ecstatic.

"I've lived with those scars for so long, I can barely remember myself without all of them," Laura says. "My skin has improved so much, it's hard to believe what a difference it makes. I no longer feel so self-conscious about how I look."

The introduction of lasers launched nothing short of a revolution in dermatology and cosmetic surgery. Lasers opened numerous treatment possibilities, either by improving existing procedures or by providing treatments for conditions that had not been treatable. Thanks to lasers, you no longer have to live with the skin conditions that accompanied you into this world, be they moles or other marks such as port-wine stains. Nor do you have to endure forever the results of a youthful enthusiasm for tattoos. Tattoos used to be difficult to remove, and attempts to erase them often left ugly scars and involved considerable recovery time. In contrast, removing tattoos with lasers is minimally invasive, although it may require five or more treatments.

As Laura experienced, the scars remaining after those long battles with acne can also be zapped by beams of laser light. Unwanted hair can be removed from the face and legs, as can vitiligo, a disfiguring autoimmune disorder that produces mottled skin with white spots—Michael Jackson is one of the most notable victims of this disease.

The key to the versatility of laser light lies in the effects different wavelengths of light have on skin tissue. The color of laser light varies according to its wavelength—there are red, green, and yellow light lasers, as well as lasers that combine colors, such as blue-green and green-yellow-red. Different colors affect skin tissue differently and are used to treat different skin conditions. Some lasers, for example, are effective on brown and red colors, so they are used to remove age spots, brown birthmarks, and red tattoos. Others work on spider veins and red or purple birthmarks, and still other lasers are effective for blue, black, and green marks, and are used to remove tattoos.

In this chapter, we review some of the most common age-related skin problems and their treatment. As you will see, in numerous cases, lasers have become one of the most important weapons in the dermatologist's arsenal. However, one size never fits all, and you are fortunate to live in a time when there are numerous treatment options for conditions that your mother simply had to live with.

Adult-Onset Acne

Although usually considered to be the scourge of teens, acne can affect adults as well, and in such cases it is harder to treat. Topical remedies commonly used for teens, as well as oral antibiotics or Accutane®, are not always as effective for adults. Adult women are more affected than men, and acne can be a problem right up to menopause.

Acne occurs when dead skin cells clog up hair follicles, causing a buildup of the sebum, or oil, produced by the hair follicle. If this causes the hair follicle to become infected and inflamed, whiteheads and blackheads develop. If the follicle bursts, surrounding areas can become infected and new pimples form. The most common form of acne, *acne vulgaris* ("vulgaris" means common), affects 90 percent of adolescents and about 50 percent of adult women. Fortunately, this type of acne only causes scarring in the most severe cases. In contrast, scarring is an all-too-common outcome of cystic acne, one of the worst forms of acne, which develops when an infected pimple erupts beneath the skin and infects the surrounding tissue.

What causes adult acne is not known. In one survey, 57 percent of women sufferers attributed their acne to stress, and it is possible that stress is a contributing factor. Stress can increase the male hormone, testosterone, in both women and men, and higher levels of testosterone can lead the oil glands to produce more oil.

Cosmetic ingredients, such as oil- and petroleum-derived products, can also trigger acne outbreaks. If you tend to break out in a certain area of the face, check to see whether it is caused by a specific cosmetic product you are using in that area. In general, use only mild cosmetic products and avoid scrubbing or irritating your skin in other ways. Only use a moisturizer if you need to, and make sure it is oil-free.

Although acne generally can't be cured, there are numerous ways to reduce its symptoms and prevent scarring. Over-the-counter products often work well for fairly mild cases of acne, but you may have to try several different types before you find something that works for you. If your acne is chronic or severe, seek out medical advice to deal with the problem.

One of the most common ingredients in over-the-counter acne products is benzoyl peroxide, which has both antibacterial and drying properties and curbs acne by preventing infection and reopening clogged pores. Over-the-counter benzoyl peroxide products have fairly low concentrations and are a good place to start. If you haven't gotten results within a couple of months, get a prescription for a benzoyl peroxide product with a stronger concentration.

Salicylic acid, a beta hydroxy acid, is another over-the-counter product that may help to control acne because of its exfoliating action. By peeling off the surface skin cells, it cleanses the pores and prevents the clogging that is the first step in the formation of acne. Other over-the-counter products include astringents that dry the skin and remove dead skin cells, such as witch hazel, resorcinol (often combined with sulfur to maximize results), and isopropyl alcohol. The last is a very strong astringent and should be used only sparingly.

If over-the-counter remedies don't do anything for you, try some of the many topical acne remedies or oral medications available by prescription only. Tretinoin products such as Retin-A and Micro Retin-A can be extremely effective. Topical and oral antibiotics are also sometimes prescribed to treat the symptoms of acne. Antibiotics eradicate the bacteria that infect clogged pores, reducing skin inflammation and curbing the spread of infection to surrounding tissue. It may take several weeks for improvement to occur, and the treatment often extends for longer than a year. Although oral antibiotics often produce excellent results, they may be associated with uncomfortable side effects, such as allergies, gastrointestinal problems, and sun sensitivity.

One of the most controversial oral acne medications is Accutane (the brand name for isotretinoin), used to treat severe cystic acne. Accutane curbs the skin's oil production and prevents dead skin cells from clogging pores. Although Accutane produces excellent results, it should be used with caution. It has been known to produce severe side effects, including vision problems, depression, and elevated cholesterol. It should never be used during pregnancy, as it may cause birth defects.

Hormonal therapy can also be effective at controlling acne. Hormonal imbalances are indicated if outbreaks typically occur in the week before a woman gets her period. Hormone treatment particularly benefits women in their twenties and thirties who have a history of menstrual irregularities, premenstrual acne outbreaks, and facial oiliness. The treatment uses oral contraceptives or antiandrogens, which block the effects of testosterone (androgen) on oil glands and hair follicles. The result is a reduction in oil production and reduced outbreaks. Improvement frequently occurs within a month and usually within two or three months.

Most acne treatments require prolonged care, from months to years. Once improvement is achieved, a maintenance dose is usually necessary. In severe cases, some form of treatment may be necessary until menopause. Early research suggests that some lasers may be helpful treating inflammatory acne.

Acne scars can be treated in a variety of ways, depending on the type of scarring. Because of the great versatility they offer in treating different types of scars, lasers are increasingly the treatment of choice. Many of the lunchtime lasers produce excellent results with no downtime, but multiple treatments are needed to produce results. Deeper resurfacing lasers, such as the Er:YAG and CO_2, often require as little as one treatment. For best results, a combination of treatments may be required.

A more traditional method of treating acne scars is dermabrasion, which uses a rotary instrument to "sand" down or abrade the skin. Since scars are depressions in the skin, the treatment works by lowering the surrounding skin so the scar is no longer visible. Nowadays, dermabrasion and other methods of treating acne scars, such as moderate chemical peels, are used less frequently.

Microdermabrasion can be used to remove very mild acne scarring. For more severe scarring, a surgical procedure known as excision and punch replacement graft is sometimes used. During this procedure, a depressed acne scar is removed, and a patch of skin from elsewhere on the body is grafted on to the scar. In cases of severe scarring from cystic acne, autologous fat transfer can be used. As discussed earlier, fat is taken from the body and injected below the surface of the skin in the area of the scarring. The effect is to elevate the depressed scar to the same level as the rest of the skin. Results last from six to eighteen months, and multiple procedures can make the gains permanent. As an alternative to the person's own fat, bovine collagen, collagen-related fillers, and other implants may be used.

If you are taking Accutane, you must discontinue the medication for at least six to twelve months before a laser treatment, because Accutane interferes with the healing process. If you will have follow-up treatments, you should also avoid taking Accutane in the intervening period. You can continue with other acne medications, such as oral antibiotics and benzoyl peroxide. People who currently suffer from severe acne should not undergo the more aggressive laser treatments, since the ointments and dressings used after surgery can aggravate the existing condition.

Age Spots

Next to wrinkles, age spots — or liver spots as they are also sometimes called — are one of the most prevalent and unflattering signs of aging. Caused mainly by excessive sun exposure, age spots are large brown marks that look like oversized freckles. The medical term for the spots is *lentigines*, and they occur primarily on sun-exposed regions of the body, such as the face and the back of the hands.

Although a variety of topical creams have been developed to treat lentigines, none work terribly well. The best way to treat such spots is with pigment-specific Q-switched lasers. One or two treatments usually lead to dramatic results. A sunscreen with a minimum of SPF 15 should be used continuously after the age spots are removed, to reduce the development of new ones.

Cellulite

Cellulite is fatty and fibrous connective tissue that gives the skin a dimpled and puckered look. Usually found on the thighs and buttocks, it occurs mostly in women, usually after the age of thirty. Being overweight does not in itself cause cellulite; some slim women develop cellulite, while some obese women have none.

You should be wary of the many cellulite "cures" advertised. Despite enthusiastic advertising claims, no cream, potion, or lotion so far has been scientifically proven to have any effect on the condition. Cellulite is not an easy problem to treat, but some women have found improvement through an outer thigh and buttock lift. Lasers do not have any effect on cellulite, nor does liposuction.

Some women swear by a treatment known as Endermalogie®, a procedure developed in France over a decade ago. The treatment uses rollers and suctioning to massage affected areas, increasing the circulation and—so its advocates claim—breaking down fat and cellulite. The procedure is painless and feels like a deep massage. Each session takes about a half hour, but a series of treatments is necessary for visible results. If you are going to benefit from Endermalogie, you will see the results within ten sessions. Most people hit a plateau between fifteen and twenty sessions, and after that, monthly maintenance sessions are necessary. Endermalogie is not cheap; a single session can cost up to $125.

Endermalogie works best in combination with a diet and exercise program, or you may see no results at all. Despite the enthusiastic claims of its proponents, the treatment remains controversial. Some physicians argue that the effects can result from diet and exercise alone, while other physicians believe that the results are of greater magnitude than could be expected from diet and exercise alone. According to one study published in *Plastic and*

Reconstructive Surgery in 1999, women who underwent twice-weekly Endermalogie treatments exhibited no objectively measurable results. Nonetheless, ten women out of the thirty-five in the study reported that, in their subjective judgment, their cellulite had improved.

So be cautious in what to expect from this procedure; it is not guaranteed to work. Your best bet for preventing or reducing cellulite is also the least expensive: stick to a good diet and maintain a regular exercise routine. If you find it hard to muster the discipline to exercise, consider using the money you might otherwise spend on expensive cellulite treatments to hire a personal trainer to get you started — even if you can only afford a few sessions. Once you get going, you'll find it easier to keep up a good exercise routine on your own.

Dark Circles under the Eyes and Baggy Lower Eyelids

Dark circles under the eyes can be a real problem, because they typically make you look tired and older than you are. There are many causes of this condition. It often develops when the skin under the eyes becomes thinner and more transparent with age. As a result, the blood in the fine veins under the eyes makes the skin appear darker. In people with dark skin, such as those of Mediterranean descent, the dark circles may also be due to superficial pigmentation of the skin in that area.

Although dark circles under the eyes are not necessarily an indication that you are not getting enough sleep, insomnia or sleep deprivation sometimes does play a role. Lack of sleep may cause the veins under the eyes to fill with more blood, which darkens the skin in that area. Fatigue can also cause the muscles to relax or lose tone. In addition, in people who suffer from allergies, hay fever, or asthma, the fine veins under the eyes often become congested, contributing to dark circles. Less common causes of dark circles include pregnancy, which can cause hormonal changes that lead to the condition, and birth control pills, which may increase pigmentation under the eyes.

Sometimes the dark circles are just a shadow cast by bags below the eyes. As we age, the fat that protects the eyeball relocates slightly, which may create a small fat bulge underneath the eyes. The groove beneath the fat bulge looks like a dark circle. Bags under the eyes can also be caused by fluid retention, which although mostly harmless, can be an indicator of serious health problems, such as high blood pressure, or heart, thyroid, kidney, or liver problems.

A number of skin creams on the market purport to treat dark circles, but there is little evidence they work. If you have dark circles under the eyes, your best bet is to work with a dermatologist who can help you pinpoint the cause of the condition and develop the best treatment strategy. If the dark circles are due to swelling and fluid retention, something as simple as applying cool tea bags or cool cucumber slices under the eyes may bring relief.

For people with dark skin, where dark circles are due to superficial skin pigmentation, lightening agents can help, although they must be used with great care on the sensitive skin under the eye. Some physicians also recommend Intense Pulsed Light or laser treatments to reduce prominent pigmentation under the eyes and remove dark circles.

If the dark circles are caused by shadows cast by bags under the eyes, the treatment of choice is a cosmetic eyelid surgery called *blepharoplasty*. During this procedure, excess skin and fat pads under the eyes are removed. Once the fat bulges beneath the eyes are gone, the dark circles automatically disappear. Discomfort is mild, and pain can be controlled by over-the-counter or prescription pain medicine. The incision heals quickly and is barely visible in two to four weeks. For best results, laser resurfacing is sometimes recommended as an adjunct to blepharoplasty if there are a lot of wrinkles around the eyes.

Melasma

Melasma is a brown discoloration occurring especially on the cheeks, nose, and chin. Unlike age spots, which present as isolated brown spots, melasma shows up as blotchy, irregular patches of excess pigmentation. The condition is most prevalent among women of childbearing age and it is most commonly caused by sun damage or hormonal influences. Genetic predisposition also plays a role; the condition is most widespread among women with skin types III and IV, such as Asian-Americans and people of Mediterranean descent.

Melasma often develops during pregnancy or in women who use oral contraceptives. Some researchers believe it is induced when estrogen stimulates the pigment-producing cells in the skin to secrete more pigment. It's a good idea to keep an eye out for melasma during high-risk times, such as pregnancy, because the condition responds best to treatment directly following onset. If you develop melasma while taking birth control pills, you need to discontinue them to improve the condition.

Although melasma can be difficult to remove completely, a variety of topical treatments can produce improvement. The first stop is an easy one: use sunscreens religiously. Once melasma has developed, exposure to sunlight will perpetuate the condition and counteract any other treatment you might apply. Use SPF 15 or higher sunscreens that block both UVB and UVA radiation.

Skin-lightening creams are usually the treatment of choice for melasma. The most common skin-lightening agent used in these products is hydroquinone, which lightens the skin by inhibiting melanin synthesis. Hydroquinone products with a concentration of 2 percent or less are available over the counter, but these are not as effective as prescription products, which typically have concentrations of around 4 percent. Although higher concentrations of hydroquinone produce even better results, they also carry increased risk of side effects, including skin irritation, allergic reactions, and — paradoxically — hyperpigmentation in the form of dark spots.

Tretinoin preparations are also often used to treat melasma. Studies have found, for example, that treatment with a 0.1 percent tretinoin preparation over a twenty-four-week period leads to significant improvement. Although the pathways are not entirely understood, tretinoin appears to promote pigment loss in the epidermis.

In addition, treatment with alpha hydroxy acids is sometimes used, typically in the form of glycolic acid peels. The glycolic acid peel causes mild stinging and, if used in higher concentrations, redness and peeling. Although such peels are safe on most dark skin types, in rare cases, scarring and hyper- or hypopigmentation may result. Other promising agents include kojic acid and azelaic acid. Azelaic acid is derived from cereal grains; it lightens the skin by inhibiting the activity of tyrosinase, an enzyme involved in pigment production. In addition, mandelic acid, an alpha hydroxy acid derived from bitter almonds, may be helpful in fading melasma.

Best results are generally achieved by combining hydroquinone treatment with other agents, such as tretinoin and alpha hydroxy acids. Both tretinoin and AHAs may facilitate the penetration of hydroquinone into the skin, enhancing its effectiveness. For most melasma treatments, it is necessary to adopt a long-term perspective. It may take up to two months to see any results, and treatment typically needs to continue for up to a year. Use of sunscreens should be continued indefinitely to avoid recurrence.

Rosacea

Rosacea is a skin condition that causes persistent redness of the cheeks, nose, and central forehead. It is usually seen in fair-skinned adults who have a history of blushing or flushing, but it can affect people of any skin type. A common symptom is redness that looks like a sunburn but does not go away, and a burning, stinging, or tingling sensation of the affected skin. Rosacea can also show up as small, red pimples and is often confused with acne. In its more advanced stage, rosacea can trigger the appearance of spider veins, or *telangiectasias* — broken red or purple capillaries that appear in a weblike pattern on the cheeks or nose.

Rosacea-like symptoms can be caused by other ailments, so consult with a dermatologist to confirm the diagnosis if you suspect you may have rosacea. Although there is no cure for the condition, a dermatologist can help you develop a treatment plan to minimize the symptoms and prevent the condition from getting worse. Treatment can help to reduce skin redness and inflammation and prevent permanent damage. If left untreated, rosacea may develop into permanent red skin with dilated blood vessels, and, in rare cases, into a condition known as *rhinophyma*, in which the nose looks swollen and red. This problem is more common in men — the most famous sufferer of this condition was comedian W. C. Fields.

A first step in reducing rosacea outbreak is to eliminate lifestyle factors that may exacerbate the condition. Avoid alcohol, spicy foods, prolonged sun exposure, and anything that can irritate the skin, such as rubbing or harsh cosmetics and soaps.

To bring the condition under control and reduce redness and pimples, your dermatologist may start you on a combination of oral and topical antibiotics. While oral antibiotics cannot be used over the long term, topical treatment may have to be continued even after the symptoms have disappeared to prevent future flare-ups.

It should be noted that some acne treatments, such as those containing benzoyl peroxide, can worsen rosacea symptoms.

If rosacea is left untreated, spider veins or telangiectasias often develop. Lasers have proven highly successful in addressing this problem; they treat the condition by selectively targeting the enlarged blood vessels and clearing the redness (see the section below on spider and varicose veins). Intense Pulsed Light treatments are also emerging as a promising treatment for these symptoms.

Spider Veins and Varicose Veins

Some 80 million Americans suffer from unsightly blood vessels on their legs, a condition that becomes increasingly common with age. The offenders are of two types—spider veins and varicose veins. *Spider veins* are small dilated blood vessels located close to the surface of the skin; they appear to be a web of red or purple lines. Also referred to as telangiectasias or broken capillaries, spider veins can develop on the legs and the face. Although spider veins on the face sometimes are a symptom of rosacea, the condition can also result from genetic predisposition, sun damage, pregnancy and childbirth, injury, estrogen replacement therapy, or use of corticosteroids.

Varicose veins are enlarged blood vessels that have become distended as a result of weakness in the vein wall, which causes the vessel to widen and inflate. Varicose veins appear only on the legs, and they differ from spider veins in a number of ways. They are larger and tend to bulge or twist; they are darker in appearance, with a red, purple, or bluish tint; and they are located deeper than spider veins. Varicose veins are often painful, and where spider veins are primarily a cosmetic concern, varicose veins can pose health risks. Because the vein does not provide an adequate supply of oxygen or fluid drainage from the skin, the surrounding skin may develop ulcers, or the vein itself may become inflamed or develop blood clots.

Spotlight on Research

NEW TREATMENT FOR VASCULAR LESIONS
In a study involving two hundred patients, IPL therapy was used to treat a wide range of red facial blemishes, including prominent facial veins (primarily telangiectasias, other symptoms of rosacea, and port-wine stains). Subjects received one to four treatments, depending on the severity of their problem. At two months' follow-up, more than 90 percent of the subjects who returned exhibited 75 to 100 percent improvement. No subject developed scarring or other permanent side effects. The researchers concluded that IPL therapy may address problems that are resistant to laser therapy, with a minimum of discomfort.

Women are four times as likely as men to suffer from varicose veins. According to the American Society for Dermatologic Surgery, 41 percent of women between the ages of forty and fifty suffer from varicose veins, and the number increases to a whopping 72 percent of women age sixty to seventy. With age, the veins also become more visible and pronounced.

The best cure for varicose veins is prevention. While heredity does play a role, the problem is exacerbated by numerous lifestyle factors, such as excess weight and a sedentary lifestyle. In addition, excessively tight clothing and stockings that restrict circulation in your legs can provoke the condition, as can uncomfortable, high-heeled shoes. Varicose veins also develop in response to changes in hormonal levels brought about by pregnancy, menopause, or use of birth control pills.

Walking regularly is a simple and effective way to prevent varicose veins and reduce existing ones. Walking tones your muscles, improves the circulation in your legs, and, over time, reduces your body weight. Also, take ten- to fifteen-minute breaks several times during the day and put your legs up to take pressure off them. Compression stockings can help to control symptoms and prevent the condition from progressing. Available at most pharmacies, these stockings concentrate pressure near the ankles, helping to push blood upward and reducing the pressure on the veins.

For years, the primary form of treatment for spider veins and varicose veins was a needle injection technique known as sclerotherapy. During this procedure, a sclerosing (hardening) solution is injected into the vein. The irritation caused by the solution makes the vein collapse, and the body reabsorbs it over time.

Several vessels are typically injected during a treatment session, and a vessel usually has to be injected more than once during several treatment sessions spaced four to six weeks apart. Although sclerotherapy is safe when performed by an experienced physician, it can be painful and may create bruises and brown streaks in the injected areas immediately after the procedure. These are a normal part of the process and generally disappear over time. Less common side effects include hard lumps, redness, or open sores.

Another treatment, known as the closure technique, bombards the vein with radio frequency energy through a small catheter placed inside the vein, causing the vein wall to shrink and close down. As the vein dies off, healthier veins in the surrounding tissue take over and restore normal blood flow to the area. This technique can be quite useful for larger spider veins.

The advent of lasers and IPL technology has introduced less invasive ways of treating spider veins and small varicose veins. Smaller surface veins respond particularly well to IPL treatments during which the vein is exposed to intense light energy. When absorbed by the blood, the light creates enough heat to destroy the vein. Recently developed laser treatments have also provided effective and relatively painless ways of treating both spider veins and some varicose veins. Precisely targeted laser light is used to heat the blood in the vein, which makes the blood coagulate. The coagulated blood vessels shrink in size and gradually fade away as they are eliminated naturally by the body's immune system. Since the laser light is absorbed only by the blood vessels, normal skin is left unharmed, reducing the risk of scarring and recurrence of the spider or varicose veins.

Several laser treatments over a period of time may be necessary to provide maximal lightening or complete removal of the veins. Depending on the severity of the condition and the depth of the veins, different types of lasers are used. Your doctor will decide which type will work best for your situation.

In one study we co-authored, presented at the American Society for Laser Medicine and Surgery meeting in New Orleans in 2001, treatment of spider veins with an Nd:YAG laser produced significant improvement in 71 percent of twenty-one subjects ages twenty-two to sixty-nine.

Laser treatment for spider or varicose veins involves little discomfort, and you can typically return to normal activity immediately after treatment. In most cases, all you will feel is a sunburn-like sensation that lasts for several hours. Sometimes a blue-black bruise appears immediately after treatment that may last seven to ten days. Some patients develop a slight brown discoloration at the treatment site as the blood vessels are absorbed into the body. If discoloration does develop, it can be expected to fade over time.

Stretch Marks

Stretch marks are the pink or violet lines that appear as the skin stretches during pregnancy, rapid growth, or weight gain. They are usually found on the breasts, thighs, and abdomen. Over time, the redness fades, but the depressed marks remain.

Before the advent of lasers, the only treatment available for stretch marks was daily application of a topical cream containing tretinoin (Retin-A). This can be a somewhat messy process that frequently requires six to twelve months before any improvement is seen.

If stretch marks are of recent onset, laser treatment can be quite effective. It produces improvement after only one or two treatments, even though additional treatments are sometimes required to obtain maximal results. Our most recent research, presented at the annual conference of the American Society for Lasers in Surgery and Medicine in April 2002, indicates that laser surgery can also make older stretch marks less noticeable. The treatments were done with an excimer laser on women with stretch marks on their thighs, upper arms, or buttocks. Most patients had six to nine treatments, each lasting five to ten minutes. The stretch marks became less noticeable in all of the women, and the marks kept their repigmentation when they were checked after six months. However, the laser did not change the texture, indentations, or other aspects of stretch marks.

An alternative to laser treatment might be a "tummy tuck," which can be effective for stretch marks below the navel, since the procedure removes much of the skin in that area.

Unwanted Hair

While unwanted and unflattering hair growth often develops as early as puberty, it can emerge at later stages of life as well — during pregnancy or menopause, or with the use of certain medications, including hormones, birth control pills, and certain blood pressure medicines. Growth of unwanted or excess hair is most often caused by hormonal changes or genetic or ethnic factors, not by an undetected medical problem or condition.

Special Considerations for Ethnic Skin

Laser technology has created a number of ways to eliminate hair problems common among people of African-American descent. Some 12 million African-American men in the United States are affected by "barber's itch," or shaving bumps. The medical term for this condition is *pseudofolliculitis barbae,* and it develops if shaved hair curls back and grows back into the skin, causing inflammation and local scarring. The long-pulsed Nd:YAG laser has been used with great success to prevent this condition by removing facial hair. Two other conditions that respond well to laser treatments are *hidradenitis suppurativa* and *dissecting cellulitis.* These conditions occur in many skin types, but they are particularly prevalent among people with black skin. Both are diseases of the hair follicle that create pimplelike lesions and abscesses prone to infection and scarring. Traditional treatment has been topical and oral antibiotics to curb the inflammation, but laser hair removal is becoming a preferred means of preventing or slowing down the disease by zapping away at-risk hair follicles.

For temporary removal of unwanted or excess hair, epilation is one of the most commonly used techniques. Epilation is just a fancy word for standard hair removal methods, such as shaving, waxing, or tweezing, that either cut off the hair or pull the hair shaft out from the follicle. Another technique, depilation, uses a strong chemical solution to destroy the hair. Both of these methods provide only a temporary solution, since hair regrowth occurs as soon as one to four weeks in most cases.

Until recently, electrolysis was the only treatment available to provide permanent hair removal. This treatment uses electricity to destroy the hair follicle: a fine needle is inserted down each individual hair follicle, one at a time, and an electric current is turned on to destroy the hair. The technique is time-consuming, costly, and often painful, and it is inefficient for treating large areas of excess hair growth, such as the back, legs, or bikini line.

The introduction of lasers for removing unwanted hair was a watershed event, in that it vastly improved the ease and effectiveness with which unwanted hair can be removed permanently. The treatment was controversial when it was first developed in the mid-1990s, but it is now accepted. It rivals electrolysis in the successful treatment of small hairy areas, and surpasses anything else in treatment of larger areas.

The newest laser procedures deliver short, powerful pulses of light to treat the hair-bearing skin. In addition to the laser, a specialized handpiece incorporates a chiller device that is held against the skin during laser exposure. Cool water or a cold spray flows from the handpiece to reduce discomfort and protect the skin from injury during delivery of the laser light.

Extensive clinical research has shown that the laser light is selectively and precisely absorbed by the brown melanin pigment found in the hair shaft and the reproductive cells of the hair follicle responsible for producing new hairs. The duration of the short pulse of light from the laser is carefully designed to disable the hair follicle without excessively heating the skin surrounding it. Absorption of laser light by these pigmented structures heats the hair follicle cells and damages them sufficiently to hinder hair regrowth.

This technique is capable of quickly and effectively removing hair from small anatomic sites, like the area above the lip, and large areas, like the back and legs. If large or sensitive areas with excess or unwanted hair are treated, it may be advisable to apply a topical anesthetic cream to the treatment site to reduce discomfort. In most cases, however, this is not necessary.

It is impossible to know in advance how many treatments will be needed, because the laser only disables hairs that are in their active growth phase at the time of treatment. Since hairs in a given area are likely to have entered their growth cycles at different times, retreatment is necessary to disable all the hair follicles. While occasional patients have long periods of no hair growth after a single laser treatment, it is more likely that more treatments will be necessary.

CHAPTER 13

Getting Old
Can Be Beautiful

*T*he increase in life expectancy that we have witnessed over the last hundred years is nothing less than astounding. Thanks to improvements in public health, advances in medicine, and enhanced living conditions, the average person today will live some thirty years longer than a hundred years ago. Such an increase in life expectancy is unprecedented in human history, and science is still catching up to the new needs and demands created by the increased proportion of the population that lives well beyond age fifty.

The more than 77 million aging baby boomers now entering middle age will be the largest cohort ever to enjoy this extended life expectancy. By the year 2030, close to every fourth person in the United States will be over age sixty-five. As maturing boomers look for new ways to counteract the assaults of aging, they are scooping up anti-aging drugs and cosmetics to the tune of more than $30 billion a year—a number expected to grow to $41.9 billion by 2006.

If one is to believe the enthusiastic advertising claims, greater energy, a more youthful appearance, and reversal of age-related afflictions can be yours simply by spending a few (or sometimes not so few) dollars on testosterone therapy, human growth hormone supplementation, or high-potency antioxidant supplements with miraculous, life-extending properties. Still, as alluring as the many promises of extended youth are, it is advisable to proceed with caution. The claims for many of these products and substances often have little basis in scientific reality or may misrepresent the science behind them. In many cases, using such products may amount at best to throwing money out the window, or at worst, they can have an adverse impact on your health and longevity—the exact opposite of what you are trying to achieve. As we saw in chapter 6, for example, some hormones, such as estrogen and progesterone, can indeed counteract some of the physiological changes associated with aging. Even so, however, estrogen supplementation is associated with other, undesirable effects, some of which may even be life-threatening. When it comes to supplementation with other hormones, such as human growth hormone or testosterone, the story may be no different. Although there is some evidence that these may have some benefits (when they are administered under supervision of medical professionals), this does not automatically mean that supplementation with these hormones will enhance your health and longevity. Indeed, recent studies on animals indicate that regular intake of growth hormone, for example, might in fact shorten life span.

When it comes to supplementation with megadoses of antioxidants or vitamins, there is also reason for caution. The fact that a given nutrient has benefits when ingested as part of a normal, healthy diet does not automatically mean that these benefits can be magnified by ingesting it in large doses in supplement form.

Beta-carotene is a well-known case in point. This important antioxidant is thought to play a key role in preventing a number of chronic diseases that become more prevalent with age, including cancer, stroke, and heart disease. Unfortunately, ingesting large doses of beta-carotene in supplement form may have adverse health consequences.

The bottom line is that there is no simple, magical shortcut to retaining youthful energy and appearance. As we have seen throughout this book, this does not mean that you have no choice but to throw up your hands and let nature take its course. All other things being equal, it is within your power to increase your chances of living a long, full, and happy life and to extend the period of time in which you are in full bloom. The simple acts of eating a healthy diet, getting enough exercise, and balancing your activity to minimize stress and tension can do more for your ability to enjoy the second half of your life than anything else.

In short, the most important person in the unfolding of the aging process as it pertains to your own body and mind is you. No external treatment, no matter how effective, can attain as much for your general long-term health, well-being, and appearance as the simple act of taking good care of your body. The downside of increased life expectancy and advances in medical care is that many people will spend a larger proportion of their lives being sick. By some estimates, the average person living in today's society will be sick 10 percent of his or her life, having to endure such chronic diseases as osteoporosis, cancer, Alzheimer's, arthritis, or heart disease. If your search for the key to retaining a youthful appearance leads you to adopt more healthy lifestyle practices that can prevent such diseases, instead of simply shelling out money for easy external "fixes," you will be ahead of the game. By adopting simple preventive activities and avoiding unhealthy behaviors such as smoking, excessive eating, or alcohol consumption, not only will you improve your vitality and energy, you will also maximize your chances of enjoying better health as you grow older. And it is never too late to improve your health, fitness, and overall appearance.

In addition, it makes a lot of sense to do what you can to mask the signs of aging by availing yourself of the many breakthrough therapies and treatments described in this book. Dramatic advances in laser surgery and the promise of the emerging science of cosmeceuticals are among the most encouraging developments to come along on the anti-aging scene for a while. In particular, if you are one of the many people who wince at the thought of having to undergo cosmetic surgery, these developments are good news for you. Nonablative laser treatments and related technologies such as Intense Pulsed Light therapy have introduced far more sophisticated tools for counterbalancing the ravages of aging than have been available in the past. Because these treatments stimulate the skin's own regenerative processes and increase youthfulness from the inside out, it is now possible to attain a more youthful appearance without having to resort to painful cosmetic surgery. Cosmetic surgery will continue to fulfill needs that are not met by more newly developed treatments. As a general tool for rejuvenating one's appearance in an effortless and generally painless way, however, the power of nonablative laser surgery and other technologies that work by stimulating regeneration of the deeper layers of skin tissue is unparalleled.

In fact, we may be witnessing only the beginning of a vast transformation in the knowledge and tools available for caring for maturing skin. With the increasing demands of an aging population, the quest for new and revolutionary treatments is ongoing. Progress within the field of cosmetic dermatology over the past five years has been nothing short of astonishing, and it shows no sign of slowing down. Thermalift and coblation are just two of the new arrivals on the scene, and more technologies will be developed over the next few years.

As the seasons of your life unfold, it is our wish for you that the knowledge and treatments described in this book will help you extend your youthfulness and vitality and bless you with a gracefully maturing appearance. Then, as the storms of life mellow into evening's glow, you may find that getting older has its own rewards—increased wisdom, maturity, and calm. If you are among the lucky people who reach this special place, you will find that growing old is not something to be dreaded or avoided, but in its own right, something truly beautiful.

Resources

USEFUL ORGANIZATIONS

American Academy of Anti-Aging Medicine
2415 N. Greenview Avenue
Chicago, IL 60614
1-773-528-4333
www.worldhealth.net

American Academy of Dermatology
(General information and resources for finding
a dermatologist)
930 East Woodfield Road
Schaumburg, IL 60173
1-888-462-DERM
www.aad.org

American Council on Exercise
4851 Paramount Drive
San Diego, CA 92123
1-800-825-3636
www.acefitness.org

American Dietetic Association
216 W. Jackson Boulevard
Chicago, IL 60606
1-800-877-1600
www.eatright.org

American Society for Dermatologic Surgery
  5550 Meadowbrook Drive, Suite 120
  Rolling Meadows, IL 60008
  1-847-956-0900
  Consumer hotline: 1-800-441-2737
  www.asds-net.org

American Society for Laser Medicine and Surgery
  2404 Stewart Square
  Wausau, WI 54401
  1-715-845-9283
  www.aslms.org

FDA Center for Food Safety and Applied Nutrition
  5100 Paint Branch Parkway
  College Park, MD 20740
  1-888-SAFEFOOD
  www.cfsan.fda.gov

HELPFUL WEBSITES

American Dietetic Association Home Page
  Information about everything from the latest nutritional
  research to how to find a dietitian to advise on achieving
  specific health goals
  www.eatright.org

American Academy of Dermatology Online Education
  An online educational resource of the American Academy
  of Dermatology
  www.skincarephysicians.com/agingskinnet/index.html

Arbor Nutrition Guide
  A comprehensive source of links to dietary information
  on the web
  http://arborcom.com

Cosmeticscop
Useful, consumer-oriented information about skin care and
cosmetics products
www.cosmeticscop.com

FDA Center for Food Safety and Applied Nutrition
Information about cosmetics ingredients, labeling guidelines
www.cfsan.fda.gov/~dms/cos-toc.html

Food and Nutrition Information Center
Lists food and nutrition topics from A to Z
www.nal.usda.gov/fnic/etext/fnic.html

MedlinePlus Health Information/Physical Fitness
General information and advice on how to enhance physical
fitness
www.nlm.nih.gov/medlineplus/exercisephysicalfitness.html

Bibliography

Altemus M, Rao B, Dhabhar FS, Ding W, Granstein RD. Stress-induced changes in skin barrier function in healthy women. *J Invest Dermatol*. 2001;117:309-17.

Angermeier MC. Treatment of facial vascular lesions with intense pulsed light. *J Cutan Laser Ther*. 1999;1:95-100.

Bailey AJ. Molecular mechanisms of ageing in connective tissues. *Mech Ageing Dev*. 2001; 122:735-55.

Bailey AJ, Paul RG, Knott L. Mechanisms of maturation and ageing of collagen. *Mech Ageing Dev*. 1998;106:1-56.

Benedetto AV. The environment and skin aging. *Clin Dermatol*. 1998;16:129-39.

Bergeret-Galley C, Latouche X, Illouz YG. The value of a new filler material in corrective and cosmetic surgery: DermaLive and DermaDeep. *Aesthetic Plast Surg*. 2001;25:249-55.

Bisonnette R, Allas S, Moyal D, Provost N. Comparison of UVA protection afforded by high sun protection factor sunscreens. *J Am Acad of Dermat*. 2000; 43:1036-8.

Blatt T, Mundt C, Mummert C, Maksiuk T, Wolber R, Keyhani R, et al. [Modulation of oxidative stresses in human aging skin]. *Z Gerontol Geriatr*. 1999;32:83-8.

Brincat M, Moniz CF, Studd JW, Darby AJ, Magos, A. Cooper D. Sex hormones and skin collagen content in postmenopausal women. *Br Med J*. 1983; 287(6402):1337-8.

Brincat MP. Hormone replacement therapy and the skin. *Maturitas.* 2000; 35:107-117.

Brzezinski A, Debi A. Phytoestrogens: The 'natural' selective estrogen receptor modulators. *Eur J Obstet Gynecol Reprod Biol.* 1999; 85:47-51.

Callens A, Vaillant L, Lecomte P, Berson M, Gall Y, Lorette G. Does hormonal skin aging exist? *Dermatology.* 1996;193:289-94.

CE.R.I.E.S. (CEntre de Recherches et d'Investigations Epidermiques et Sensorielles) of Chanel. Signs of Aging Skin. Dossier de Presse, 1998.

Darr D, Dunston S, Faust H, Pinnell S. Effectiveness of antioxidants (vitamin C and E) with and without sunscreens as topical photoprotectants. *Acta Derm Venereol.* 1996;76:264-8.

DeBuys HV, Levy SB, Murray JC, Madey DL, Pinnell SR. Modern Approaches to Photoprotection. *Dermatol Clin.* 2000;18:577-90.

Dreher F, Maibach H. Protective effects of topical antioxidants in humans. *Curr Probl Dermatol.* 2001;29:157-64.

Etcoff N. *Survival of the Prettiest.* New York, NY. Anchor Books; 2000.

Fitzpatrick RE, Rostan EF. Double-blind, half-face study comparing topical vitamin C and vehicle for rejuvenation of photodamage. *Dermatol Surg.* 2002;28:231-6.

Giacomoni PU, Rein G. Factors of skin ageing share common mechanisms. *Biogerontology.* 2001;2:219-29.

Goldberg DJ. Nonablative subsurface remodeling: clinical and histologic evaluation of a 1320-nm Nd:YAG laser. *J Cutan Laser Ther.* 1999;1:153-7.

Goldberg DJ. Laser treatment of vascular lesions. *Clin Plast Surg.* 2000;27:173-80, ix.

Goldberg DJ. New collagen formation after dermal remodeling with an intense pulsed light source. *J Cutan Laser Ther.* 2000;2:59-61.

Goldberg DJ. Full-face nonablative dermal remodeling with a 1320 nm Nd:YAG laser. *Dermatol Surg.* 2000;26:915-8.

Goldberg DJ. Laser hair removal. *Dermatol Clin.* 2002;20:561-7.

Goldberg DJ. Laser treatment of pigmented lesions. *Dermatol Clin.* 1997;15:397-407.

Goldberg DJ. Nonablative dermal remodeling: does it really work? *Arch Dermatol.* 2002;138:1366-8.

Goldberg DJ. Nonablative resurfacing. *Clin Plast Surg.* 2000;27:287-92, xi.

Goldberg DJ. Nonablative subsurface remodeling: clinical and histologic evaluation of a 1320-nm Nd:YAG laser. *J Cutan Laser Ther.* 1999;1:153-7.

Goldberg DJ. Unwanted hair: evaluation and treatment with lasers and light source technology. *Adv Dermatol.* 1999;14:115-39; discussion 140.

Goldberg DJ, Arndt KA. Is a medical degree necessary to perform laser and surgical procedures? *Dermatol Surg.* 2000;26:85-6.

Goldberg DJ, Cutler KB. The use of the erbium:YAG laser for the treatment of class III rhytids. *Dermatol Surg.* 1999;25:713-5.

Goldberg DJ, Cutler KB. Nonablative treatment of rhytids with intense pulsed light. *Lasers Surg Med.* 2000;26:196-200.

Goldberg DJ, Marcus J. The use of the frequency-doubled Q-switched Nd:YAG laser in the treatment of small cutaneous vascular lesions. *Dermatol Surg.* 1996;22:841-4.

Goldberg DJ, Meine JG. Treatment of facial telangiectases with the diode-pumped frequency-doubled Q-switched Nd:YAG laser. *Dermatol Surg.* 1998;24:828-32.

Goldberg DJ, Meine JG. A comparison of four frequency-doubled Nd:YAG (532 nm) laser systems for treatment of facial telangiectases. *Dermatol Surg.* 1999;25:463-7.

Goldberg DJ, Rogachefsky AS, Silapunt S. Nonablative laser treatment of facial rhytides: a comparison of 1450-nm diode laser treatment with dynamic cooling as opposed to treatment with dynamic cooling alone. *Lasers Surg Med.* 2002;30:79-81.

Goldberg DJ, Samady JA. Evaluation of a long-pulse Q-switched Nd:YAG laser for hair removal. *Dermatol Surg.* 2000;26:109-13.

Goldberg DJ, Samady JA. Intense pulsed light and Nd:YAG laser nonablative treatment of facial rhytids. *Lasers Surg Med.* 2001;28:141-4.

Goldberg DJ, Silapunt S. Q-switched Nd:YAG laser: rhytid improvement by nonablative dermal remodeling. *J Cutan Laser Ther.* 2000;2:157-60.

Goldberg DJ, Whitworth J. Laser skin resurfacing with the Q-switched Nd:YAG laser. *Dermatol Surg.* 1997;23:903-6; discussion 906-7.

Gorman C, Park A. The truth about hormones. *Time;* July 22, 2002:33-39.

Gray J. *The World of Skin Care. A Scientific Companion.* London, England: Macmillan Press, Ltd, 2000.

Greenwood-Robinson M. *Wrinkle-Free. Your Guide to Youthful Skin at Any Age.* New York, NY: Berkley Books; 2001.

Han KK, Soares JM Jr, Haidar MA, de Lima GR, Baracat EC. Benefits of soy isoflavone therapeutic regimen on menopausal symptoms. *Obstet Gynecol.* 2002;99:389-94.

Harris ED, Rayton JK, Balthrop JE, DiSilvestro RA, Garcia-de-Quevedo M. Copper and the synthesis of elastin and collagen. *Ciba Found Symp.* 1980;79:163-82.

Hoppe U, Bergemann J, Diembeck W, et al. Coenzyme Q10, a cutaneous antioxidant and energizer. *Biofactors.* 1999;9:371-8.

Knuutinen A, Kokkonen N, Risteli J, et al. Smoking affects collagen synthesis and extracellular matrix turnover in human skin. *Br J Dermatol.* 2002;146:588-94.

Koblenzer C. Psychologic aspects of aging and the skin. *Clin Derm.* 1996;14:171-177.

Krol ES, Kramer-Stickland KA, Liebler DC. Photoprotective actions of topically applied vitamin E. *Drug Metab Rev.* 2000;32:413-20.

Lawrence N. New and emerging treatments for photoaging. *Dermatol Clin.* 2000;18:99-112.

Liu J, Burdette JE, Xu H, Gu C, van Breemen RB, Bhat KP, et al. Evaluation of estrogenic activity of plant extracts for the potential treatment of menopausal symptoms. *J Agric Food Chem.* 2001;49:2472-9.

Liu S, Willett WC. Dietary glycemic load and atherothrombotic risk. *Curr Atheroscler Rep.* 2002;4:454-61.

Lu LJ, Tice JA, Bellino FL. Phytoestrogens and healthy aging: gaps in knowledge. A workshop report. *Menopause.* 2001;8:152-3.

Lucas EA, Wild RD, Hammond LJ, et al. Flaxseed improves lipid profile without altering biomarkers of bone metabolism in post-menopausal women. *J Clin Endocrinol Metab.* 2002; 87:1527-32.

McVean M, Liebler DC. Inhibition of UVB induced DNA photo-damage in mouse epidermis by topically applied alpha-toco-pherol. *Carcinogenesis.* 1997;18:1617-22.

Nusgens BV, Humbert P, Rougier A, et al. Topically applied vita-min C enhances the mRNA level of collagens I and III; their pro-cessing enzymes and tissue inhibitor of matrix metallopro-teinase 1 in the human dermis. *J Invest Dermatol.* 2001;116:853-9.

Parentini L. *The Joy of Healthy Skin. A Lifetime Guide to Beautiful Problem-Free Skin.* Englewood Cliffs, NJ: Prentice Hall; 1996.

Perricone NV, Topical 5% alpha-lipoic acid cream in the treat-ment of cutaneous rhytids. *Aesthetic Surg J.* 2000; 218-222.

Perugini P, Genta I, Pavanetto F, Conti B, Scalia S, Baruffini A. Study on glycolic acid delivery by liposomes and micros-pheres. *Int J Pharm.* 2000;196:51-61.

Pierard GE, Letawe C, Dowlati A, Pierard-Franchimont C. Effect of hormone replacement therapy for menopause on the mechanical properties of skin. *J Am Geriatr Soc.* 1995;43:662-5.

Pinnell SR, Yang H, Omar M, et al. Topical L-ascorbic acid: per-cutaneous absorption studies. *Dermatol Surg.* 2001;27:137-42.

Polnikorn N, Goldberg DJ, Suwanchinda A, Ng SW. Erbium:YAG laser resurfacing in Asians. *Dermatol Surg.* 1998; 24:1303-7.

Pozner JM, Goldberg DJ. Histologic effect of a variable pulsed Er:YAG laser. *Dermatol Surg.* 2000;26:733-6.

Preuss HG. Effects of glucose/insulin perturbations on aging and chronic disorders of aging: the evidence. *J Am Coll Nutr.* 1997;16:397-403.

Purba MB, Kouris-Blazos A, Wattanapenpaiboon N, Lukito W, Rothenberg EM, Steen BC, et al. Skin wrinkling: can food make a difference? *J Am Coll Nutr.* 2001;20:71-80.

Purba MB, Kouris-Blazos A, Wattanapenpaiboon N, et al. Can skin wrinkling in a site that has received limited sun exposure be used as a marker of health status and biological age? *Age Ageing.* 2001;30:227-34.

Ridges L, Sunderland R, Moerman K, Meyer B, Astheimer L, Howe P. Cholesterol lowering benefits of soy and linseed enriched foods. *Asia Pac J Clin Nutr.* 2001;10:204-11.

Rogachefsky AS, Silapunt S, Goldberg DJ. Nd:YAG laser (1064 nm) irradiation for lower extremity telangiectases and small reticular veins: efficacy as measured by vessel color and size. *Dermatol Surg.* 2002;28:220-3.

Rogachefsky AS, Silapunt S, Goldberg DJ. Evaluation of a new super-long-pulsed 810 nm diode laser for the removal of unwanted hair: the concept of thermal damage time. *Dermatol Surg.* 2002;28:410-4.

Roizen MF. *Real Age – Are You As Young As You Can Be?* New York, NY: Cliff Street Books; 1999.

Smith WP. Epidermal and dermal effects of topical lactic acid. *J Am Acad Dermatol.* 1996; 35(3 Pt 1):388-91.

Teikemeier G, Goldberg DJ. Skin resurfacing with the Erbium:YAG laser. *Dermatol Surg.* 1997;23:685-7.

Traikovich SS. Use of topical ascorbic acid and its effects on photodamaged skin topography. *Arch Otolaryngol Head Neck Surg.* 1999;125:1091-8.

Yaar M, Gilchrest BA. Skin aging. Postulated mechanisms and consequent changes in structure and function. *Clin Geriatr Med.* 2001;17:617-30.

Index